the
Zucchini
Spiralizer
Cookbook

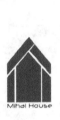

Mihai House

the Zucchini Spiralizer Cookbook

Zucchini Spaghetti Maker Recipes for
Tasty Gluten-free Spiralizer Cooking - Use with Paderno,
Veggetti, Noodle & Pasta Maker

Kari James

DISCLAIMER

ISBN-13: 978-1508813576
ISBN-10: 1508813574

CONTENTS

13
EASY CONVERSION GUIDE 231

1

MORE ZOODLES PLEASE

E ver just wished you had more recipe ideas for your spiralized zucchini noodles? Then, welcome to the spiralizer cookbook of zucchini recipes! Now, you can add more fun to your spiralizer cooking with a book that specially features the all-time favorite and easiest spiralizable vegetable. The zucchini! Everyone loves to make zucchini spaghetti, it's just like that. So whether you call it squash, courgette, summer squash or just plain old zucchini, you'll love this spiralizer cookbook.

This cookbook serves up over 100 delectable and interesting spiralized zucchini recipes that everyone can make to support a healthy lifestyle. More specifically, the nutrient-dense zoodle recipes in this book may be used for:

- Gluten-Free Diet
- Paleo Diet
- Weight Loss Diet
- Low Carb Diet
- Dairy-Free Diet
- Low Calorie Diet
- High Fiber Diet

Interestingly, even though the peak season for zucchinis is between May and July, zucchinis have been well known for their abundance all year round. Despite their abundance, home cooks would quickly become tired of preparing zucchini the same old boring ways over and over again. But thanks to the spiralizer! Now, we can all say goodbye to the once boring and bland zucchini meals and welcome a whole new world of exciting and creative zucchini cooking. Yes! This cookbook is nicely organized with more than enough delightful recipes that will give your zucchini dishes the ultimate makeover.

You don't have to be an experienced cook to be able to cook these zoodle recipes. Instead, the recipes consist of simple ingredients and directions that are friendly for home cooks just like you. Additionally, you won't find the politics of different spiralizers in this cookbook—it's just about cooking sumptuous zucchini pasta recipes with whichever spiralizer you own. Besides, most (if not all) spiralizers can do a zucchini.

WHY YOU NEED TO EAT MORE SPIRALIZED ZUCCHINIS

Many people are totally unaware of the rich health benefits of the zucchini. However, zucchinis are among one of the healthiest vegetables and could be referred to as one of nature's super foods. Apart from the rich nutrients and fiber that are present in zucchinis, here are some other reasons why you should start eating more:

1. **Zucchinis are good for bone health.** Zucchinis contain large amounts of bone strengthening nutrients such as magnesium and phosphorous. Copper and manganese are also present in zucchinis which will also contribute to a healthy bone metabolism. This is great news for people who

suffer from or people who are at risk of osteoporosis.

2. **Zucchinis are low in calories and carbs.** One cup of spiralized zucchini contains only 36 calories! This makes them perfect for those who are seeking to consume fewer calories or lose weight. Thumbs up for weight loss! Additionally, you could cut carbs by up to 70 percent if you make a switch from regular pasta to zucchini pasta.

3. **Zucchinis are easy to spiralize.** You simply wash your zucchini then use a sharp knife to evenly chop off both ends. Then evenly chop the zucchini in half and process with your spiralizer according to manufacturer's instructions.

4. **Zucchinis can be prepared very quickly.** Zucchinis can be eaten raw or cooked. A bowl of spiralized zucchinis is basically ready to eat as it is or it can be sautéed with a little olive oil, salt and pepper in as little as 3 minutes. That's fast!

5. **Zucchinis are good for eye health.** Zucchinis are rich in Vitamin A. This makes it a very good vegetable for optimum eye health.

6. **Zucchinis are good for our immune system.** You can boost your immune system with the abundance of Vitamin C and E in zucchinis.

7. **Zucchinis help to fight cancer.** Antioxidant rich zucchinis are great for warding off cancer and harmful free radicals in the body.

8. **Zucchinis are good for heart health.** Due to the rich combination of magnesium and potassium in zucchinis, they are good for lowering blood pressure, maintaining healthy cholesterol levels and contributing to overall heart health.

Ultimately, by increasing your zucchini consumption you will also be providing your body with essential nutrients and fiber for better health. Also, the more zucchinis you eat, the more you'll be able to maintain your optimum body weight. So, if you would simply switch from eating regular pasta to spiralized zucchini pasta, you'll be amazed at the health results.

2

HOW TO USE THIS COOKBOOK

*A*fter you have chosen a recipe, you should follow the specific recipe directions. Even though all recipes contain spiralized zucchinis, for creativity and nutritional balance, you may also find other spiralized vegetables in a few recipes. You should always use your spiralizer model according to the manufacturer's instructions. Additionally, for ease of use and a healthy variety, this book is conveniently organized into eight (8) recipe categories:

1. **EGG RECIPES** – here you'll find a variety of spiralized zucchini noodles combined with eggs and other nutritious ingredients. Some of these recipes are perfect for healthy spiralized zucchini breakfast ideas.

2. **MEATLESS RECIPES** – here you'll find a variety of spiralized zucchini noodles combined other nutritious ingredients that do not include meat. Some of these recipes may be perfect for meat-free ideas or vegans.

3. **POULTRY RECIPES** – here you'll find a variety of spiralized zucchini noodles combined with chicken or turkey ingredients. Some of these recipes may be perfect for dinner or lunch.

4. **BEEF, PORK & LAMB RECIPES** – here you'll find a variety of spiralized zucchini noodles combined with meat and other healthy ingredients. Some of these recipes may be perfect for dinner or lunch.

5. **FISH & SEAFOOD RECIPES** – here you'll find a variety of spiralized zucchini noodles combined with fish and seafood ingredients. Some of these recipes may also be perfect for dinner or lunch.

6. **SAUCE RECIPES** – here you'll find a variety of spiralized zucchini noodles combined with interesting sauce ingredients. This category consists of some of the quickest and easiest to prepare recipes.

7. **HOLIDAY RECIPES** – here you'll find a variety of spiralized zucchini noodles that are used to create interesting holiday or special occasion meals.

8. **VARIETY RECIPES** – here you'll find a variety of spiralized zucchini noodles that are combined to create delectable meals with the use of nuts and other healthy ingredients.

LET'S START ZOODLING AROUND!

Whichever recipe you choose, just follow the recipe directions and you'll be amazed at how easily you can cook interesting spiralized vegetable meals. You can certainly make your own ingredient replacements to suit your personal taste or diet preferences.

Without further ado, it's time to start using your spiralizer or spiral slicer to make creative and nutritious zucchini spaghetti meals. Let's start zoodling around!

3

EGG RECIPES

Spiced Zucchini Omelet

This dish makes a quick breakfast for the whole family. The Jalapeño pepper, fresh cilantro/coriander and scallions add a delicious touch to this omelet.

MAKES: 2 servings
PREPARATION TIME: 15 minutes
COOKING TIME: 10 minutes

2 tablespoons Coconut Oil, Extra Virgin

1 small Garlic Clove, minced

2 medium Zucchinis, spiralized

Sea Salt, to taste

Freshly Ground Black Pepper, to taste

4 large Organic Eggs

½ Jalapeño Pepper, seeded and minced

2 teaspoons minced Cilantro/Coriander Leaves

⅛ teaspoon Red Pepper Flakes, crushed

2 Scallions, chopped

Directions

1. In a large skillet, heat 1 tablespoon of the oil on a medium heat. Sauté the garlic for 1 minute. Add the zucchini and a pinch of salt and black pepper and cook for 3 minutes before removing from the heat and setting aside.
2. Meanwhile, beat together the eggs, jalapeño pepper, cilantro, red pepper flakes, salt and black pepper in a bowl. In a large frying pan, heat the remaining oil on a medium heat. Add the beaten eggs and, with a wooden spoon, spread the eggs towards the edges of pan. Cook for about 1 to 2 minutes. Place the zucchini mixture and scallions over the eggs. Carefully fold the omelet in half and cook for a further 2 minutes.

Zucchini Chicken Frittata

This is a delicious frittata which will be a hit for weekend breakfasts. This dish is packed with healthy chicken, eggs and vegetables.

MAKES: 4 servings
PREPARATION TIME: 15 minutes
COOKING TIME: 42 minutes

3 tablespoons Extra Virgin Olive Oil

2 (4-ounce) Grass-Fed boneless, diced Chicken Breasts

Sea Salt, to taste

Freshly Ground Black Pepper, to taste

2-3 Garlic Cloves, minced

1 cup Shiitake Mushrooms, sliced

2 small Zucchinis, spiralized

1½ cups Fresh Spinach, chopped

8 Organic Eggs

¼ cup Parsley Leaves, freshly chopped

Directions

1. Preheat the oven to 375 degrees F. In a large oven

proof skillet, heat 2 tablespoons of the oil on a medium-high heat. Cook the chicken, sprinkled with salt and black pepper, for 4 to 5 minutes. Transfer the chicken onto a plate. Heat the remaining oil on a medium heat and sauté the garlic for about 1 minute. Add the mushrooms and cook for 4 to 5 minutes. Add the zucchini, spinach, salt and black pepper and cook for 3 to 4 minutes. Stir in cooked chicken.

2. Meanwhile, beat together the eggs, a pinch of salt and black pepper in a bowl. Pour the egg mixture into the skillet and stir well. Cook for about 1 to 2 minutes. Transfer the skillet into the oven and bake for 20 to 25 minutes. Garnish with the parsley and serve.

Zucchini with Scrambled Eggs

This is a wonderfully delicious way to use garden fresh zucchini. This recipe prepares a quick, healthy breakfast for a busy morning.

MAKES: 4 servings
PREPARATION TIME: 15 minutes
COOKING TIME: 17 minutes

2 tablespoons Extra Virgin Olive Oil

1 large Yellow Onion, chopped

2 Garlic Cloves, minced

1 teaspoon Dried Thyme, crushed

2 large Zucchinis, spiralized

2 teaspoons Fresh Lime juice

Sea Salt, to taste

Freshly Ground Black Pepper, to taste

4 Organic Eggs, beaten

2 tablespoons minced Cilantro Leaves

Directions

1. In a large skillet, heat the oil on a medium heat.

Sauté the onion for 8 to 10 minutes before adding the garlic and thyme and sautéing for 1 minute more. Add the zucchini, salt and black pepper and cook for 2 to 3 minutes before stirring in the lemon juice.

2. Stir in the beaten eggs and cook for a further 2 to 3 minutes, tossing occasionally. Garnish with the cilantro and serve hot.

Zucchini Style Fried Eggs

This healthy recipe is a great and easy way to sneak in fresh zucchini with eggs. This dish makes a super quick breakfast for those busy mornings.

MAKES: 2 servings
PREPARATION TIME: 15 minutes
COOKING TIME: 8 minutes

2 tablespoons Extra Virgin Olive Oil

1 Garlic Clove, minced

½ Jalapeño Pepper, seeded and chopped

2 large Zucchinis, spiralized

Sea Salt, to taste

Freshly Ground Black Pepper, to taste

4 Organic Eggs

Pinch of Red Pepper Flakes, crushed

2 tablespoons Parsley, freshly chopped

Directions

1. In a large skillet, heat 1½ tablespoons of the oil on a medium heat. Add the garlic and jalapeño pepper and sauté for 1 minute. Add the zucchini, salt and

black pepper and cook for 2 to 3 minutes.

2. Make a well in the center of the zucchini mixture. Pour the remaining oil into the well before carefully cracking the eggs into the well. Cover the skillet and cook for 3 to 4 minutes, or until cooked to your liking. Sprinkle the eggs with red pepper flakes, black pepper and salt. Garnish with the parsley and serve.

Zucchini, Tomato & Egg Salad

This is a great combination of zucchini, grape tomatoes and eggs with walnuts. The sweet and sour dressing makes a perfect blend of flavors in this garden fresh salad.

MAKES: 2 servings
PREPARATION TIME: 20 minutes

For Salad:

3 medium Zucchinis, spiralized

½ cup Grape Tomatoes, halved

¼ cup Red Onion, chopped

2 Organic Hard Boiled Eggs, peeled and chopped

1 tablespoon Scallion Leaves, freshly chopped

1 tablespoon Mint Leaves, freshly chopped

2 tablespoons Walnuts, toasted and chopped

For Dressing:

2 tablespoons Fresh Lime juice

2 tablespoons Extra Virgin Olive Oil

1 tablespoon Organic Honey

¼ teaspoon Red Pepper Flakes, crushed

Sea Salt, to taste

Freshly Ground Black Pepper, to taste

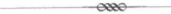

Directions

1. In a large serving bowl, mix together all of the salad ingredients, except for the walnuts. In another bowl, beat together all of the dressing ingredients. Combine the dressing with the salad and gently toss to mix.
2. Garnish with the walnuts and serve immediately.

Beefy Zoodle Casserole

This is a healthy casserole of zucchini, ground beef and eggs packed with delicious flavors. This casserole will be a perfect hit any time of the day.

MAKES: 4 servings
PREPARATION TIME: 15 minutes
COOKING TIME: 55 minutes

3 tablespoons Coconut Oil, Extra Virgin

1 small Yellow Onion, chopped

2 Garlic Cloves, minced

½ teaspoon Dried Rosemary, crushed

½ pound Grass-Fed Lean Ground Beef

3 large Zucchinis, spiralized

Sea Salt, to taste

Freshly Ground Black Pepper, to taste

¼ teaspoon Red Pepper Flakes, crushed

4 Large Eggs

½ cup Fresh Chives, chopped

Directions

1. Preheat the oven to 350 degrees F and grease a casserole dish.
2. In a large skillet, heat the oil on medium heat. Sauté the onion for 2 to 3 minutes before adding the garlic and rosemary and sautéing for 1 minute more. Add the beef and cook for 6 to 8 minutes, or until golden brown. Add the zucchini, salt and black pepper and cook for 2 to 3 minutes.
3. Meanwhile, beat together the eggs, red pepper flakes and a pinch of salt in a bowl. Pour the egg mixture into the skillet and stir well. Immediately transfer the mixture into the prepared casserole dish and bake for 35 to 40 minutes. Garnish with the chives and serve.

Zucchini, Avocado & Egg Salad

This is a fantastic recipe of a fresh, healthy and delicious salad.
This dish will be a perfect hit for lunchtime.

MAKES: 2 servings
PREPARATION TIME: 20 minutes

1 medium Zucchini, spiralized

1 medium Yellow Squash, spiralized

½ cup Black Olives, pitted and sliced

1 medium Avocado, peeled, pitted and cubed

1 teaspoon Fresh Chives, minced

2 tablespoons Parsley, freshly chopped

2 tablespoons Fresh Lemon juice

1 tablespoon Extra Virgin Olive Oil

Sea Salt, to taste

Freshly Ground Black Pepper, to taste

2 Organic Hard Boiled Eggs, peeled and sliced

Directions

1. In a large serving bowl, mix together the zucchini,

squash, olives, avocado, chives and parsley. Drizzle with the lemon juice and oil. Sprinkle with the salt and black pepper and gently toss to mix.

2. Top with the egg slices and serve immediately.

Zucchini Egg Drop Soup

This is one of the most soothing and comforting soup recipes you will come across. This soup is super easy to prepare yet delicious and healthy as well.

MAKES: 4 servings
PREPARATION TIME: 15 minutes
COOKING TIME: 25 minutes

2 tablespoons Extra Virgin Olive Oil

1 medium White Onion, chopped

2 Stalks Celery, chopped

4 Garlic Cloves, minced

4 cups Homemade Vegetable Broth

4 Organic Eggs, beaten

4 large Zucchinis, spiralized

½ cup Basil Leaves, freshly chopped

Sea Salt, to taste

Freshly Ground Black Pepper, to taste

Directions

1.   In a large soup pan, heat the oil on a medium heat.

Sauté the onion and celery for 9 to 10 minutes before adding the garlic and sautéing for 1 minute more. Add the broth and bring to a boil on a high heat. Reduce the heat and simmer for 5 to 10 minutes.

2. Slowly add the beaten eggs to the pan, stirring continuously. Stir in the zucchini, basil, salt and black pepper. Cook for a further 3 to 4 minutes before serving hot.

Zucchini & Chicken Egg Bowl

This is a delicious bowl of healthy and comforting soup! This dish is bursting with the healthy nutrients of chicken, fresh vegetables and eggs.

MAKES: 4 servings
PREPARATION TIME: 20 minutes
COOKING TIME: 40 minutes

2 tablespoons Extra Virgin Olive Oil

1½ pounds Grass-Fed boneless, diced Chicken Breasts

Sea Salt, to taste

Freshly Ground Black Pepper, to taste

1 small Yellow Onion, chopped

2 Carrots, chopped

2 Stalks Celery, chopped

½ cup Mushrooms, chopped

3-4 Garlic Cloves, minced

½ teaspoon Red Pepper Flakes, crushed

1 teaspoon Dried Thyme, crushed

6-8 cups Homemade Chicken Broth

4 Organic Eggs, beaten

2 medium Zucchinis, spiralized

½ cup Parsley, freshly chopped

Directions

1. In a large soup pan, heat the oil on a medium heat. Add the chicken and sprinkle with the salt and black pepper. Cook for 4 to 5 minutes, or until golden brown on all sides. Transfer the chicken onto a plate. Add the onion, celery, carrots and mushrooms to the pan and sauté for 9 to 10 minutes. Add the garlic, red pepper flakes and thyme and sauté for 1 minute more. Add the cooked chicken and broth, and bring to a boil on a high heat. Reduce the heat and simmer for 15 to 20 minutes.
2. Slowly add the beaten eggs to the pan, stirring continuously. Stir in the zucchini, parsley, salt and black pepper. Cook for a further 3 to 4 minutes before serving hot.

Tomato Sauce Zoodle Eggs

This recipe makes a comfort dish for a healthy breakfast or brunch. The spicy and flavorful tomato sauce makes a wonderful combination with the zucchini and fried eggs.

MAKES: 2 servings
PREPARATION TIME: 20 minutes
COOKING TIME: 40 minutes

---

3 tablespoons Coconut Oil, Extra Virgin

2 large Zucchinis, spiralized

Sea Salt, to taste

Freshly Ground Black Pepper, to taste

1 small White Onion, chopped

½ small Yellow Bell Pepper, seeded and chopped

½ small Red Bell Pepper, seeded and chopped

3-4 Garlic Cloves, minced

1 Jalapeño Pepper, seeded and chopped

1 teaspoon Whole Cumin Seeds

¼ teaspoon Red Pepper Flakes, crushed

¼ teaspoon Cayenne Pepper

4 cups Fresh Tomatoes, finely chopped

⅓ cup Homemade Vegetable Broth

4 large Eggs

½ cup Basil Leaves, freshly chopped

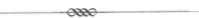

Directions

1. In a large skillet, heat 1 tablespoon of the oil on a medium heat. Add the zucchini, salt and black pepper and cook for 2 to 3 minutes. Transfer the zucchini onto a plate and set aside. Heat the remaining oil on a medium heat in the same skillet. Add the onion and bell peppers and sauté for 5 to 6 minutes. Add the garlic, jalapeño pepper and spices and sauté for 1 minute more. Add the tomatoes to the skillet and cook for 1 to 2 minutes whilst crushing with the back of a spoon. Add the broth and bring the dish to a gentle simmer. Simmer for about 20 minutes before stirring in the zucchini.
2. Make a well in the center of the zucchini mixture and carefully crack the eggs into the well. Cover the skillet and cook for 5 to 8 minutes, or until cooked to your liking. Sprinkle the eggs with salt and black pepper, garnish with the basil and serve.

Zucchini with Poached Eggs

Surprise your family with a simple yet tasty breakfast. This dish is guaranteed to delight the taste buds of your whole family!

MAKES: 2 servings
PREPARATION TIME: 10 minutes
COOKING TIME: 20 minutes

---

2 tablespoons Coconut Oil, Extra Virgin

1 Red Onion, chopped

1 Garlic Clove, minced

2 large Zucchinis, spiralized

Sea Salt, to taste

Freshly Ground Black Pepper, to taste

4 Eggs

1 large Scallion, finely chopped

Directions

1. In a large skillet, heat the oil on a medium heat. Sauté the onion for 8 to 10 minutes before adding the garlic and sautéing for 1 minute more. Add the zucchini and cook for 3 to 4 minutes. Transfer the zucchini mixture onto a large serving plate.

2. Meanwhile, in large pan, boil water on a medium-high heat. Reduce the heat to medium and crack 1 egg into a bowl. Carefully pour the egg into the pan of boiling water and repeat with the remaining eggs. Cook for 4 to 5 minutes, or until cooked to your liking. Place the poached eggs over the cooked zucchini. Sprinkle the eggs with salt and black pepper, garnish with the scallion and serve immediately.

Zucchini Egg Garden

This is a gorgeous recipe for breakfast, brunch or lunch. This dish will surely become one of your favorites.

MAKES: 4 servings
PREPARATION TIME: 20 minutes (plus time for ingredients to infuse)
COOKING TIME: 8 minutes

2 Garlic Cloves, minced and divided

4 cups Cherry Tomatoes, finely chopped

1 cup Fresh Basil Leaves, minced

2 tablespoons Fresh Lemon juice

3 tablespoons Extra Virgin Olive Oil

½ teaspoon Red Pepper Flakes, crushed and divided

Sea Salt, to taste

Freshly Ground Black Pepper, to taste

4 medium Zucchinis, spiralized

½ cup Black Olives

4 large Organic Eggs

Directions

1. In a large bowl, mix together 1 garlic clove, the cherry tomatoes, basil, lemon juice, 1 tablespoon of oil, ⅛ teaspoon of red pepper flakes, salt and black pepper. Set aside for at least 15 minutes to develop the flavors. In a large skillet, heat the remaining oil on a medium heat. Add the remainder of the garlic and sauté for 1 minute before adding the zucchini and cooking for 2 minutes. Add the olives, remaining red pepper flakes, salt and black pepper and cook for 2 minutes more. Transfer the zucchini mixture onto a large serving dish.

2. In large pan, boil water on a medium-high heat. Reduce the heat to medium and crack 1 egg in a bowl. Carefully pour the egg into the pan of boiling water and repeat with the remaining eggs. Cook for 2 to 3 minutes, or until cooked to your liking.

3. Add the tomato mixture into the dish with the zucchini mixture. Place the poached eggs over the tomato mixture and break the eggs with a spoon. Gently toss the dish and serve immediately.

4

MEATLESS RECIPES

Lemony Spiced Zucchini Salad

This is a quick, easy and delicious salad idea for a light lunch. You will love to add this recipe to your menu list.

MAKES: 2 servings
PREPARATION TIME: 15 minutes

1 large Zucchini/Courgette, spiralized

1½ tablespoons Fresh Lemon juice

1 teaspoon Ground Cumin

⅛ teaspoon Red Pepper Flakes, crushed

Sea Salt, to taste

Pinch of Freshly Ground Black Pepper

1 teaspoon Lemon Zest, freshly grated

Directions

1. Add all of the ingredients into a large serving bowl and toss to coat well.
2. Serve immediately.

Roasted Beets Zucchini Salad

This recipe is a creative and healthy twist to a simple plate of salad. The combination of spiralized zucchini and roasted beets make this creative salad really delicious.

MAKES: 4 servings
PREPARATION TIME: 15 minutes
COOKING TIME: 1 hour

2 Beets, trimmed

1 tablespoon Extra Virgin Olive Oil

Sea Salt, to taste

Freshly Ground Black Pepper, to taste

1 large Zucchini/Courgette, spiralized

2 large Carrots, peeled and spiralized

¼ cup Red Onion, chopped

1 tablespoon Coconut Vinegar

1 tablespoon Basil Leaves, freshly chopped

Directions

1. Preheat the oven to 350 degrees F and place foil paper in a baking sheet. Arrange the beets on the

43

foil paper. Drizzle with the oil and sprinkle with salt and black pepper. Fold the foil paper around beets and roast for about 1 hour. Remove the beets from the oven and let them cool before cutting the beets into bite size pieces. Transfer the beets into a large serving bowl.

2. Add the remaining ingredients into the bowl with the beets. Season with salt and black pepper and toss to coat well before serving immediately.

Zucchini Salad with Vegetables

This is a refreshingly light and crunchy spiralized zucchini and vegetable salad. The tangy vinaigrette with this salad adds a wonderfully tasty touch to this dish.

MAKES: 4 servings
PREPARATION TIME: 15 minutes
COOKING TIME: 1 hour

For Salad:

2 large Zucchinis/Courgettes, spiralized

1 cup Black Olives, pitted and sliced

1 cup Grape Tomatoes, halved

½ cup Orange Bell Pepper, seeded and thinly sliced

1 Red Onion, chopped

For Vinaigrette:

1 Garlic Clove, minced

1 tablespoon Fresh Parsley, minced

1 tablespoon Coconut Vinegar

1 tablespoon Fresh Lemon juice

1 tablespoon Extra Virgin Olive Oil

Sea Salt, to taste

Freshly Ground Black Pepper, to taste

Directions

1. Mix together all of the salad ingredients in a large bowl.
2. In another bowl, beat together all of the vinaigrette ingredients before pouring the vinaigrette over the salad. Ensure the dressing is mixed well with the salad before serving.

Coconut Zucchini Salad

This is a lovely and delicious spiralized zucchini pasta with a wonderful dressing. This salad is perfect for your dining table.

MAKES: 4 servings
PREPARATION TIME: 20 minutes

For Coconut Dressing:

½ cup Cashew nuts, soaked and drained

1 cup Coconut Flesh, chopped

1 teaspoon Fresh Ginger, chopped

1 Garlic Clove, chopped

¼ cup Coconut Water

2 tablespoons Fresh Lime juice

1 teaspoon Ground Cumin

Pinch of Red Pepper Flakes, crushed

Sea Salt, to taste

Freshly Ground Black Pepper, to taste

For Salad:

2 large Zucchinis/Courgettes, spiralized

3 Scallions, chopped

2 tablespoons Black Sesame Seeds

2 teaspoons Lime Zest, freshly grated

Directions

1. In a blender, add all of the dressing ingredients and pulse until smooth.
2. In a large serving bowl, place the zucchini and scallions. Add the dressing and mix well. Top with the sesame seeds and lime zest before serving immediately.

Creamy Zucchini Avocado Salad

This zucchini salad is guaranteed to impress your guests. This salad has a delicious creamy dressing which compliments nicely with the zucchini and cherry tomatoes.

MAKES: 4 servings
PREPARATION TIME: 15 minutes

1 cup Almond Milk

1 Avocado, peeled, pitted and chopped

1 small Garlic Clove, minced

¼ teaspoon Dried Parsley, crushed

¼ teaspoon Dried Dill Weed

Sea Salt, to taste

Freshly Ground Black Pepper, to taste

2 large Zucchinis/Courgettes, spiralized

1 cup Cherry Tomatoes, halved

¼ cup Scallions, finely chopped

Directions

1. In a blender, add the almond milk and avocado,

garlic, parsley, dill weed, sea salt and black pepper then pulse until smooth.

2. Place the zucchini, tomatoes and scallions into a large serving bowl. Add the dressing and mix well before serving immediately.

Grilled Zucchini & Tomatoes

This is an entertaining summertime spiralized zucchini recipe. This dish is a quick way to prepare a delicious meal without spending hours in the kitchen.

MAKES: 4 servings
PREPARATION TIME: 15 minutes
COOKING TIME: 9 minutes

3 large Tomatoes, cut into ½-inch pieces

2 tablespoons Extra Virgin Olive Oil

Sea Salt, to taste

Freshly Ground Black Pepper, to taste

2 large Zucchinis/Courgettes, spiralized

1 tablespoon Fresh Thyme, minced

2 tablespoons Fresh Lime juice

Directions

1. Preheat the grill to a medium-high heat and grease the grill grate. Generously coat the tomato slices with 1½ tablespoons of oil and sprinkle with salt and black pepper. Grill the tomato slices for about 4 minutes, turning once after 2 minutes. Remove from the grill and set aside in a bowl.

2. Place the zucchini on the grill pan. Drizzle with the remaining oil and sprinkle with salt and black pepper. Grill for 3 to 5 minutes, occasionally pressing them with the back of a spoon. Transfer the zucchini onto a serving plate and sprinkle with thyme. Arrange the tomato slices over the zucchini, drizzle with lime juice and serve.

Roasted Zucchini Veggie Combo

This is a fun way to enjoy a rainbow of delicious vegetables! These roasted vegetables not only taste great, they also look beautiful as well.

MAKES: 4 servings
PREPARATION TIME: 15 minutes
COOKING TIME: 20 minutes

2 medium Zucchinis/Courgettes, spiralized

1 small Sweet Potato, peeled and spiralized

1 large Carrot, peeled and spiralized

½ cup Mixed Bell Peppers (red, yellow, orange), seeded and sliced thinly

½ cup Red Onion, sliced

2 tablespoons Extra Virgin Olive Oil

3 tablespoons Fresh Lemon juice

1 tablespoon Fresh Rosemary, chopped

2 teaspoons Ground Cumin

½ teaspoon Cayenne Pepper

Sea Salt, to taste

Freshly Ground Black Pepper, to taste

Directions

1. Preheat the oven to 400 degrees F and grease a large baking sheet.
2. In a large bowl, add all of the ingredients and toss to coat well. Transfer the mixture onto the prepared baking sheet and roast for 10 minutes. Remove from the oven and toss the vegetables before roasting for a further 10 minutes.

Sautéed Spiced Zucchini

This easy and healthy recipe makes delicious zucchini. The combination of jalapeño pepper and spices adds a lovely spicy kick to this dish.

MAKES: 4 servings
PREPARATION TIME: 15 minutes
COOKING TIME: 6 minutes

1 tablespoon Extra Virgin Olive Oil

1 tablespoon Garlic, minced

1 Jalapeño Pepper, seeded and chopped

½ teaspoon Dried Oregano, crushed

4 medium Zucchinis/Courgettes, spiralized

½ teaspoon Ground Cumin

¼ teaspoon Cayenne pepper

Sea Salt, to taste

Freshly Ground Black Pepper, to taste

1 tablespoon minced Cilantro Leaves

Directions

1. In a large skillet, heat the oil on a medium heat.

Sauté the garlic, jalapeño pepper and oregano for about 1 minute. Stir in the zucchini and increase the heat to medium-high. Sprinkle with the spices and sauté for 4 to 5 minutes.

2. Transfer the sautéed zucchini onto a serving plate. Garnish with the cilantro and serve.

Sautéed Zucchini, Spinach & Olives

This is one of the quickest and easiest ways to cook vegetables for a delicious meal. A drizzling of lemon juice adds a refreshing touch to this dish.

MAKES: 4 servings
PREPARATION TIME: 15 minutes
COOKING TIME: 10 minutes

2 tablespoons Extra Virgin Olive Oil

4-5 Garlic Cloves, minced

2 large Zucchinis/Courgettes, spiralized

1½ cups Fresh Spinach, torn

¼ cup Cherry Tomatoes, halved

½ cup Black Olives, pitted and halved

2 tablespoons Parsley Leaves, freshly chopped

Sea Salt, to taste

Freshly Ground Black Pepper, to taste

2 tablespoons Fresh Lemon juice

Directions

1. In a large skillet, heat the oil on a medium heat. Sauté the garlic for about 1 minute. Add the zucchini and sauté for 3 to 4 minutes more. Add the spinach and cook for about 2 to 3 minutes.
2. Add the remaining ingredients, except for the lemon juice, and cook for a further2 to 3 minutes. Drizzle with the lemon juice and serve hot.

Mixed Zoodle Vegetables

This is a classic vegetarian dish full of delightful vegetables. The combination of vegetables with herbs and seasoning makes this a flavorful dish.

MAKES: 4 servings
PREPARATION TIME: 15 minutes
COOKING TIME: 20 minutes

1½ cups Broccoli Florets

1½ tablespoons Coconut Oil, Extra Virgin

¼ cup White Onion, chopped

3-4 Garlic Cloves, minced

1 Jalapeño Pepper, seeded and chopped

½ teaspoon Dried Thyme, crushed

1 cup Roma Tomatoes, finely chopped

1 Red Bell Pepper, seeded and thinly sliced

1 Orange Bell Pepper, seeded and thinly sliced

½ teaspoon Red Chili Powder

Sea Salt, to taste

2 medium Carrots, spiralized

2 medium Zucchinis, spiralized

2 tablespoons Fresh Lime juice

2 tablespoons Parsley Leaves, freshly chopped

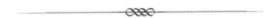

Directions

1. In a pan of boiling salted water, add the broccoli and boil for 2 to 3 minutes before draining and setting aside. In a large skillet, heat the oil on a medium heat. Sauté the onion for 3 to 4 minutes. Add the garlic, jalapeño pepper and thyme and sauté for about 1 minute. Add the tomatoes and cook, stirring, for about 2 minutes. Add the bell peppers and cook for a further 2 to 3 minutes.
2. Add the carrots and cook for about 1 to 2 minutes. Add the zucchini and cook for 2 to 3 minutes more. Stir in the broccoli, chili powder and salt and cook for 1 to 2 minutes. Stir in the lemon juice and remove from heat.
3. Garnish with the parsley and serve.

Zucchini Mushroom Splash

This is a delicious recipe that beautifully combines zucchini, eggplant, mushrooms and tomatoes. A touch of fresh dill takes this garden fresh zucchini and eggplant dish to a new level.

MAKES: 2 servings
PREPARATION TIME: 15 minutes
COOKING TIME: 16 minutes

1½ tablespoons Extra Virgin Olive Oil

2-3 Garlic Cloves, minced

3 Scallions, chopped

1 cup Portobello Mushrooms, chopped

1 cup Eggplant, cubed

2 cups Fresh Plum Tomatoes, finely chopped

½ cup Homemade Vegetable Broth

Sea Salt, to taste

Freshly Ground Black Pepper, to taste

2 large Zucchinis/Courgettes, spiralized

2 tablespoons Fresh Dill, minced

Directions

1. In a large skillet, heat the oil on a medium heat. Sauté the garlic for about 1 minute. Add the scallions and mushrooms and cook for 3 to 4 minutes. Add the eggplant and cook for 2 to 3 minutes.

2. Add the tomatoes and cook, stirring, for 1 to 2 minutes. Add the broth, black pepper and salt and bring to a boil. Cook, whilst stirring occasionally, for 2 to 3 minutes. Stir in zucchini and cook for a further 2 to 3 minutes. Stir in the dill and serve.

Zucchini Roasted Tomatoes

This is a super quick and easy to prepare meal for the whole family. This recipe will help you to prepare a delicious and healthy dish.

MAKES: 2 servings
PREPARATION TIME: 15 minutes
COOKING TIME: 11 minutes

1½ cups Grape Tomatoes

1½ tablespoons Extra Virgin Olive Oil

Sea Salt, to taste

Freshly Ground Black Pepper, to taste

1 medium Onion, chopped

2 Garlic Cloves, minced

2 large Zucchinis/Courgettes, spiralized

1 tablespoon Fresh Lemon juice

2 tablespoons Fresh Parsley, chopped

2 tablespoons Walnuts, toasted and chopped

Directions

1. Preheat the oven to 400 degrees F and line a baking

sheet with parchment paper. Place the tomatoes in the prepared baking sheet. Drizzle with ½ tablespoon of oil and sprinkle with salt and black pepper. Toss to coat well and roast for about 10 minutes. Transfer the tomatoes into a bowl and set aside.

2. In a large skillet, heat the remaining oil on a medium heat. Sauté the onion for 4 to 5 minutes before adding and sautéing the garlic for about 1 minute. Add the zucchini, black pepper and salt and cook, whilst stirring occasionally, for about 5 minutes. Stir in the lemon juice and parsley and remove from the heat.

3. Transfer the zucchini mixture onto a serving plate. Place the roasted tomatoes over the zucchini mixture, top with the walnuts and serve.

Zucchini Broccoli Zest

This recipe makes a simply light yet hearty dish. This dish will be a great choice for the menu at lunchtime.

MAKES: 2 servings
PREPARATION TIME: 15 minutes
COOKING TIME: 25 minutes

12-14 Broccoli Florets

2 large Garlic Cloves, minced and divided in half

2 tablespoons Fresh Lime juice

2 tablespoons Extra Virgin Olive Oil

Sea Salt, to taste

Freshly Ground Black Pepper, to taste

1 Jalapeño Pepper, seeded and chopped

2 large Zucchinis/Courgettes, spiralized

½ teaspoon Lime Zest, freshly grated

Directions

1. Preheat the oven to 420 degrees F and grease a baking sheet. In a large bowl, mix together the broccoli, half of the minced garlic cloves, lime juice,

1 tablespoon of oil, salt and black pepper. Roast for about 15 to 20 minutes. Transfer the broccoli mixture into a bowl and set aside.

2. In a large skillet, heat the remaining oil on a medium heat. Add the remaining garlic and jalapeño pepper and sauté for about 1 minute. Add the zucchini, salt and black pepper and cook, whilst stirring occasionally, for 3 to 4 minutes. Stir in the broccoli mixture and remove from the heat. Garnish with lime zest and serve.

Spicy Zucchini & Mushroom Stew

This spicy and delicious stew, made with zucchini noodles and mushrooms is ideal for a light meal.

MAKES: 2 servings
PREPARATION TIME: 15 minutes
COOKING TIME: 10 minutes

---

1 tablespoon Coconut Oil, Extra Virgin

½ teaspoon Fresh Ginger, minced

2 Garlic Cloves, minced

1 Lemongrass Stalk, chopped

1 Serrano Pepper, seeded and chopped

½ teaspoon Ground Cumin

¼ teaspoon Ground Cilantro

¼ teaspoon Turmeric Powder

¼ teaspoon Cayenne Pepper

1 cup Button Mushrooms, chopped

1 cup Cabbage, shredded

1½ cups Homemade Vegetable Broth

2 large Zucchinis/Courgettes, spiralized

½ cup Scallions, chopped

Sea Salt, to taste

Freshly Ground Black Pepper, to taste

1 tablespoon Fresh Lemon juice

1 tablespoon Fresh Parsley, chopped

Directions

1. In a large skillet, heat the oil on a medium heat. Add the ginger, garlic, lemongrass, Serrano pepper and spices, and sauté for about 1 minute. Add the mushrooms and cabbage and cook for 3 to 4 minutes.
2. Add the broth and bring to a boil. Stir in the zucchini, scallions, salt and black pepper, and cook for 4 to 5 minutes. Stir in the lemon juice and remove from the heat before garnishing with parsley and serving.

Nutty Zucchini & Asparagus

This bowl of zucchini noodles, roasted vegetable and crunchy almonds has a great touch of delicious flavors. This recipe makes a hearty meal.

MAKES: 2 servings
PREPARATION TIME: 15 minutes
COOKING TIME: 30 minutes

8-10 White Pearl Onions, soaked and peeled

¼ cup Fresh Lemon juice

8-10 Asparagus Stalks, trimmed and cut into 2-inch pieces

2 tablespoons Extra Virgin Olive Oil

1 teaspoon Dried Rosemary, crushed

¼ teaspoon Red Pepper Flakes, crushed

Sea Salt, to taste

Freshly Ground Black Pepper, to taste

2 Garlic Cloves, minced

½ Jalapeño Pepper, seeded and chopped

2 large Zucchinis/Courgettes, spiralized

2 tablespoons Almonds, toasted and chopped

1 tablespoon Fresh Scallion, chopped

Directions

1. Preheat the oven to 375 degrees F and grease a roasting pan. In a bowl, mix together the pearl onion and lemon juice. Transfer the onions into the prepared baking dish. In another bowl, mix together the asparagus and 1 tablespoon of oil. Transfer the asparagus into the baking dish with the onions. Sprinkle with rosemary, red pepper flakes, salt and black pepper. Roast for about 25 minutes, turning once after 13 minutes.

2. In a large skillet, heat the remaining oil on a medium heat. Sauté the garlic and jalapeño pepper for about 1 minute. Add the zucchini, salt and black pepper and cook, whilst stirring occasionally, for 3 to 4 minutes. Transfer the zucchini into a serving bowl. Place the roasted asparagus and pearl onions over the zucchini. Top with the almonds and fresh scallions and serve.

5

POULTRY RECIPES

Zapara Chicken Salad

This zucchini, asparagus and grilled chicken, with a creamy avocado dressing is a perfect way to enjoy a light and refreshing meal. This is one of the best refreshing salads for summer.

MAKES: 4 servings
PREPARATION TIME: 20 minutes (plus time to marinate)
COOKING TIME: 12 minutes

For Salad:

1 teaspoon Dried Rosemary, crushed

½ teaspoon Ground Cumin

¼ teaspoon Ground Cilantro

½ teaspoon Ground Turmeric

Sea Salt, to taste

Freshly Ground Black Pepper, to taste

2 (6-ounce) Grass-Fed boneless Chicken Thighs

16 Baby Asparagus Spears, trimmed

½ tablespoon Extra virgin Olive Oil

2 large Zucchinis, spiralized

½ cup Cherry Tomatoes, halved

For Dressing:

1 small Avocado, peeled, pitted and chopped

½ small Cucumber, peeled and chopped

1 Garlic Clove, chopped

¼ cup Fresh Basil Leaves

2 tablespoons Coconut Milk

1 tablespoon Fresh Lemon juice

Sea Salt, to taste

Freshly Ground Black Pepper, to taste

Directions

1. Preheat the grill to medium-high and grease the grill grate. In a bowl, mix together the rosemary and spices. Add the chicken thighs and generously rub

with the spice mixture. Set aside for 10 minutes. Grill the thighs for 4 to 5 minutes per side, or until cooked. Remove the thighs from the grill and set aside for 5 minutes. With a sharp knife, cut the chicken thighs into your desired size slices. Transfer the chicken onto a plate.

2. Drizzle the asparagus with the oil and sprinkle with salt and black pepper. Grill the asparagus for about 2 minutes. Cut the asparagus into 2-inch pieces and place in a large serving bowl. Add the zucchini into the bowl with the asparagus.

3. For the dressing, place all of the dressing ingredients into a food processor and pulse until smooth. Mix the dressing with the salad before topping with the chicken slices. Garnish with the cherry tomatoes and serve immediately.

Green Zoodles Chicken Salad

This salad is filled with lots of bold flavors and lot of fresh crunch! This delicious dish is not only healthy; it is also accompanied with a great tasting tangy vinaigrette.

MAKES: 4 servings
PREPARATION TIME: 20 minutes (plus time to marinate)
COOKING TIME: 20 minutes

For Salad:

2 Garlic Cloves, minced

2 tablespoons Coconut Oil, Extra Virgin

½ tablespoon Coconut Aminos

1 tablespoon Fresh Lime juice

Sea Salt, to taste

Freshly Ground Black Pepper, to taste

2 (6-ounce) Grass-Fed boneless, cubed Chicken Breasts

2 medium Zucchinis, spiralized

5-6 cups Fresh Baby Greens

½ cup Pecans, toasted and chopped

For Vinaigrette:

2 tablespoons Shallots, minced

1 tablespoon Capers, finely chopped

1 Garlic Clove, minced

1 Jalapeño Pepper, seeded and minced

2 tablespoons minced Cilantro Leaves

1 teaspoon Lime Zest, freshly grated

¼ cup Extra Virgin Olive Oil

2 teaspoons Coconut Vinegar

2 tablespoons Fresh Lime juice

Sea Salt, to taste

Freshly Ground Black Pepper, to taste

Directions

1. Preheat the oven to 350 degrees F and line a baking sheet with aluminum foil. In a large bowl, mix together the garlic, oil, coconut aminos, lime juice, salt and black pepper. Add the chicken cubes and generously coat with the mixture. Set aside for 15 to 20 minutes. Transfer the mixture into the prepared baking sheet and bake for 15 to 20 minutes. Transfer the chicken cubes into a large serving bowl. Add the zucchini and greens.

2. In another medium bowl, beat together all of the ingredients for the vinaigrette before pouring the vinaigrette over the salad and tossing to coat well.

Top with the pecans and serve immediately.

Sweet & Sour Chicken Salad

This recipe is a great way of using fresh zucchini from your garden. The mildly sweet and sour dressing adds a wonderfully delicious flavor to the chicken and zucchini.

MAKES: 2 servings
PREPARATION TIME: 20 minutes
COOKING TIME: 10 minutes

For Salad:

1 tablespoon Coconut Oil, Extra Virgin

1 (6-ounce) Grass-Fed boneless Chicken Breast

Sea Salt, to taste

Freshly Ground Black Pepper, to taste

1 large Zucchini, spiralized

1 large Carrot, spiralized

2 tablespoons Mint Leaves, freshly chopped

2 tablespoons Cashew nuts, chopped

For Dressing:

1 Garlic Clove, minced

½ teaspoon Fresh Ginger, minced

1 Jalapeño Pepper, seeded and minced

2 tablespoons Coconut Cream

1 tablespoon Almond Butter

½ tablespoon Raw Honey

1 tablespoon Coconut Aminos

1 tablespoon Fresh Lemon juice

Sea Salt, to taste

Freshly Ground Black Pepper, to taste

Directions

1. In a skillet, heat the oil on a medium heat. Add the chicken and sprinkle with the salt and black pepper. Cook for 4 to 5 minutes on both sides until the chicken is cooked. Transfer the chicken onto a large plate and let it cool completely before shredding the chicken and transferring into a large serving bowl. Add the zucchini, carrot and mint.
2. In another bowl, mix together all of the ingredients for the dressing before pouring the dressing over the salad and gently mixing. Top with the cashews and serve.

Zucchini Chicken Soup

This recipe makes one of the most delicious, healthy and super easy soups to prepare.

MAKES: 4 servings
PREPARATION TIME: 10 minutes
COOKING TIME: 25 minutes

4 cups Homemade Chicken Broth

2 cups Grass-Fed cooked and shredded Chicken

2 medium Carrots, peeled and finely chopped

2 Stalks Celery, chopped

2 large Zucchinis, spiralized

Sea Salt, to taste

Freshly Ground Black Pepper, to taste

¼ cup Basil Leaves, freshly chopped

Directions

1. In a large soup pan, add the broth and bring to a boil on a high heat. Add the cooked chicken, carrots and celery. Reduce the heat and simmer for 15 to 20 minutes.
2. Stir in the zucchini, salt, black pepper and basil, and

simmer for a further 4 to 5 minutes before serving hot.

Mushroom & Chicken Zoodles

This chicken, mushroom and zucchini soup is not only mouthwatering and beautiful, it is super healthy too. This dish is a sure winner.

MAKES: 4 servings
PREPARATION TIME: 15 minutes
COOKING TIME: 45 minutes

---

2 tablespoons Extra Virgin Olive Oil

1 medium White Onion, chopped

2 medium Carrots, peeled and chopped

1½ cups Portobello Mushrooms, chopped

1 teaspoon Dried Oregano, crushed

½ teaspoon Ground Cumin

½ teaspoon Cayenne Pepper

5 cups Homemade Chicken Broth

3 cups Grass-Fed cooked and shredded Chicken

1 medium Zucchini, spiralized

1 medium Yellow Squash, spiralized

Sea Salt, to taste

Freshly Ground Black Pepper, to taste

2 tablespoons Fresh Lime juice

¼ cup Parsley Leaves, freshly chopped

Directions

1. In a large soup pan, heat the oil on a medium heat. Add the onion, carrots and mushrooms and sauté for 4 to 5 minutes. Add the oregano and spices and sauté for about 1 minute. Add the chicken and broth and bring to a boil. Reduce the heat and simmer for 30 to 35 minutes.
2. Stir in the zucchini, yellow squash, salt and black pepper and cook for a further 3 to 4 minutes. Stir in the lemon juice and parsley and immediately remove from the heat before serving hot.

Chicken Meatball Soup

This is an awesome recipe for a filling and delicious soup. The dried herbs and spices add a nice depth of flavor to this meatball and zucchini soup.

MAKES: 4 servings
PREPARATION TIME: 20 minutes
COOKING TIME: 35 minutes

For Meatballs:

¾ pound Grass-Fed Lean Ground Chicken

1 medium Organic Egg, beaten

½ teaspoon Ground Cumin

Sea Salt, to taste

Freshly Ground Black Pepper, to taste

For Soup:

1 tablespoon Extra Virgin Coconut Oil

1 small Yellow Onion, chopped

2 small Carrots, peeled and chopped

3 Stalks Celery, chopped

3-4 Garlic Cloves, minced

½ teaspoon Dried Rosemary, crushed

½ teaspoon Dried Basil, crushed

½ teaspoon Ground Cumin

¼ teaspoon Red Pepper Flakes, crushed

¼ teaspoon Cayenne Pepper

5 cups Homemade Chicken Broth

1 large Fresh Tomato, finely chopped

2 medium Zucchinis, spiralized

Sea Salt, to taste

Freshly Ground Black Pepper, to taste

¼ cup minced Cilantro Leaves

1 Avocado, peeled, pitted and chopped

Directions

1. In a large bowl, mix together all of the meatball ingredients. Make your desired sized balls from the mixture and set aside.
2. In a large soup pan, heat the oil on a medium heat. Sauté the onion, carrots and celery for 6 to 8 minutes. Add the garlic, herbs and spices and sauté for about 1 minute. Add the tomatoes and cook for 1 to 2 minutes. Add the broth and bring to a boil and cook for about 5 minutes. Add the meatballs and reduce the heat to low and simmer for about 15 minutes.
3. Stir in the zucchini, salt and black pepper and cook for 3 to 4 minutes. Stir in the cilantro and immediately remove from the heat. Garnish the

soup with avocado and serve hot.

Swedes Zucchini Chicken Salad

This is a great recipe for a lunchtime menu. The sweet and sour flavoring in this dish gives an extra bonus to the stir fried chicken and spiralized zucchini.

MAKES: 4 servings
PREPARATION TIME: 15 minutes
COOKING TIME: 13 minutes

1 tablespoon Coconut Oil, Extra Virgin

2-3 Garlic Cloves, minced

1 pound Grass-Fed boneless Chicken Thigh strips

1 tablespoon Coconut Aminos

½ tablespoon Fresh Lime juice

½ tablespoon Coconut Vinegar

½ tablespoon Raw Honey

2 large Zucchinis, spiralized

Sea Salt, to taste

Freshly Ground Black Pepper, to taste

¼ cup Parsley Leaves, freshly chopped

1 tablespoon Black, toasted Sesame Seeds

Directions

1. In a large skillet, heat the oil on a medium heat. Sauté the garlic for about 1 minute. Add the chicken and stir fry for 2 to 3 minutes. Add the coconut aminos, lime juice, vinegar and honey, and cook for 4 to 5 minutes.

2. Stir in the zucchini, salt and black pepper and cook for a further 3 to 4 minutes. Stir in the parsley and immediately remove from the heat. Garnish with the sesame seeds and serve hot.

Zucchini Spinach Deal

This recipe makes a dish that is crammed with healthy nutrients. It is filling and full of flavorful herbs and other ingredients.

MAKES: 2 servings
PREPARATION TIME: 15 minutes
COOKING TIME: 20 minutes

6-ounces Grass-Fed boneless Chicken Breast strips

1 tablespoon Fresh Rosemary, minced

Sea Salt, to taste

Freshly Ground Black Pepper, to taste

1 tablespoon Extra Virgin Olive Oil

1 Garlic Clove, minced

2 cups Spinach, freshly chopped

2 medium Zucchinis, spiralized

½ tablespoon Fresh Lime juice

Directions

1. Preheat the oven to 350 degrees F and grease a baking dish. Arrange the chicken strips in the prepared baking dish. Sprinkle with the rosemary,

salt and black pepper, and bake for 15 to 20 minutes before removing from the oven and setting aside.

2. Meanwhile, in a skillet, heat the oil on a medium heat. Sauté the garlic for about 1 minute. Add the spinach and cook for 2 to 3 minutes. Add the zucchini, salt and black pepper and cook for a further 3 to 4 minutes. Stir in the chicken and lime juice and remove from the heat before serving hot.

Spicy Zoodles & Tomatoes

The spiralized zucchini makes a delicious combination with the chicken, tomatoes and spices in this wonderful dish. This recipe is guaranteed to be a hit with the whole family.

MAKES: 2 servings
PREPARATION TIME: 15 minutes
COOKING TIME: 30 minutes

1 tablespoon Extra Virgin Olive Oil

2 (4-ounce) Grass-Fed boneless Chicken Breasts

Sea Salt, to taste

Freshly Ground Black Pepper, to taste

⅓ cup White Onion, chopped

2 cups Tomatoes, chopped

½ teaspoon Ground Cumin

¼ teaspoon Ground Cilantro

¼ teaspoon Cayenne Pepper

½ cup Homemade Chicken Broth

2 medium Zucchinis, spiralized

2 tablespoons Thyme, freshly chopped

Directions

1. In a large skillet, heat the oil on a medium heat. Add the chicken and sprinkle with salt and black pepper. Cook for about 3 to 4 minutes before turning and cooking for 4 to 5 minutes on the other side. Add the onion and sauté for 4 to 5 minutes. Add the tomatoes and spices and cook for 1 to 2 minutes more whilst crushing the tomatoes with the back of a spoon. Add the broth and bring to a boil before reducing the heat and simmering for 10 minutes.

2. Add the zucchini, salt and black pepper and cook for a further 3 to 4 minutes. Stir in the thyme and remove from the heat before serving hot.

Zucchini Chicken & Broccoli

This recipe makes a complete meal which is really delicious. The brilliant red cherry tomatoes, green broccoli and zucchini turn these chicken thighs into a colorful meal.

MAKES: 4 servings
PREPARATION TIME: 15 minutes
COOKING TIME: 25 minutes

2 tablespoons Coconut Oil, Extra Virgin

1 Garlic Clove, minced

1 pound Grass-Fed boneless, cubed Chicken Thighs

Sea Salt, to taste

Freshly Ground Black Pepper, to taste

1 medium Yellow Onion, chopped

3 cups Broccoli florets, chopped

2 cups Cherry Tomatoes, halved

2 large Zucchinis, spiralized

½ teaspoon Red Pepper Flakes, crushed

2 tablespoons Fresh Lime juice

Directions

1. In a large skillet, heat 1 tablespoon of the oil on a medium heat. Sauté the garlic for about 1 minute. Add the chicken and sprinkle with the salt and black pepper. Cook for 6 to 8 minutes before transferring the chicken onto a plate.

2. In the same skillet, heat the remaining oil on a medium heat. Sauté the onion for 6 to 7 minutes. Add the broccoli and tomatoes and cook for 4 to 5 minutes. Stir in the zucchini, red pepper flakes, salt and black pepper, and cook for a further 3 to 4 minutes. Stir in the chicken and lime juice and remove from heat before serving hot.

Zucchini Chicken Casserole

The simple and delicious ingredients come together nicely in this flavor-packed casserole. This creamy casserole features zucchini, mushrooms and chicken.

MAKES: 4 servings
PREPARATION TIME: 20 minutes
COOKING TIME: 45 minutes

¼ cup Coconut Oil, Extra Virgin

1½ pounds Grass-Fed boneless Chicken Breast strips

Sea Salt, to taste

Freshly Ground Black Pepper, to taste

½ cup White Onion, chopped

2 cups Mushrooms, sliced

3-4 Garlic Cloves, minced

1 tablespoon Fresh Rosemary, chopped

½ cup Coconut Cream

½ cup Homemade Chicken Broth

2 tablespoons Fresh Lemon juice

6 medium Zucchinis, spiralized

1 cup Almond Meal

¼ cup Basil Leaves, freshly chopped

2 tablespoons Almonds, chopped

Directions

1. Preheat the oven to 375 degrees F and lightly grease a casserole dish.
2. In a large skillet, heat 2 tablespoons of the oil on a medium heat. Add the chicken and sprinkle with the salt and black pepper. Cook for 4 to 5 minutes before transferring the chicken onto a plate. Add the onion and mushroom to the skillet and sauté for 3 to 4 minutes. Add the garlic and rosemary and sauté for 1 minute more. Add the coconut cream, broth and lemon juice and bring to a boil before reducing the heat and simmering for 5 minutes until the sauce has thickened. Remove the skillet from the heat and stir in the chicken, zucchini, salt and black pepper. Transfer the mixture into the prepared casserole dish.
3. In a bowl, add the almond meal, remaining oil and some salt. Using your hands, mix the mixture until crumbly. Evenly spread the almond meal mixture over the zucchini mixture. Bake for 25 to 30 minutes. Garnish with basil and chopped almonds before serving.

Zucchini Chicken Stew

This medley of chicken, zucchini, bell peppers and tomatoes makes for a perfect stew for a cold winter's day. The use of fresh tomatoes gives this filling and hearty stew a full texture.

MAKES: 4 servings
PREPARATION TIME: 15 minutes
COOKING TIME: 50 minutes

2½ tablespoons Extra Virgin Olive Oil

2½ pounds Grass-Fed Chicken, cut into desired pieces

Sea Salt, to taste

Freshly Ground Black Pepper, to taste

1 large White Onion, chopped

1 medium Red Bell Pepper, seeded and cut into thin strips

1 medium Orange Bell Pepper, seeded and cut into thin strips

1 large Carrot, peeled and thinly sliced

2 Garlic Cloves, minced

2 Serrano Peppers, seeded and chopped

2 cups Fresh Tomatoes, finely chopped

2 cups Homemade Chicken Broth

2 large Zucchinis, spiralized

¼ cup minced Cilantro Leaves

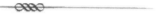

Directions

1. In a large skillet, heat 2 tablespoons of the oil on a medium heat. Add the chicken and sprinkle with salt and black pepper, and cook for 10 to 15 minutes. Transfer the chicken onto a large plate. Add the onion, bell peppers and carrots to the skillet and sauté for 3 to 4 minutes. Add the garlic and Serrano peppers and sauté for 1 minute. Add the tomatoes and cook for 1 to 2 minutes more whilst crushing the tomatoes with the back of a spoon. Add the broth and chicken and bring to a boil before reducing the heat and simmering for 20 to 25 minutes.
2. Add the zucchini, salt and black pepper and cook for a further 2 to 3 minutes. Stir in the cilantro and remove from the heat before serving hot.

Veggie Spaghetti & Meatballs

This dish is a great idea for a healthy and delicious meal. This recipe is a great dish to let your kids eat vegetables in a delicious and fun way.

MAKES: 4 servings
PREPARATION TIME: 15 minutes
COOKING TIME: 30 minutes

For Meatballs:

1 cup Carrot, peeled and roughly chopped

1 cup Zucchini, roughly chopped

3-4 Garlic Cloves, chopped

½ cup Scallion Leaves, chopped

1 Jalapeño Pepper, seeded and chopped

1 pound Grass-Fed boneless Chicken Breasts

1 Organic Egg

¼ cup Blanched Almond Flour

Sea Salt, to taste

Freshly Ground Black Pepper, to taste

For Pesto:

1 cup Fresh Basil

2 cups Fresh Baby Spinach

4 Garlic Cloves, chopped

1 tablespoon Fresh Lime juice

3 tablespoons Extra Virgin Olive Oil

Sea Salt, to taste

Freshly Ground Black Pepper, to taste

For zucchini:

2 tablespoons Extra Virgin Olive Oil

1 Garlic Clove, minced

1 Serrano Pepper, seeded and chopped

2 Medium Zucchinis, spiralized

Sea Salt, to taste

Freshly Ground Black Pepper, to taste

Directions

1. Preheat the oven to 350 degrees F and line a baking sheet with parchment paper. For the meatballs, add the carrot, zucchini, garlic, scallion and jalapeño pepper to a food processor and pulse until finely chopped. Add the remaining meatball ingredients to the food processor and pulse until combined. Make

your desired sized balls from the mixture. Arrange the balls in the prepared baking sheet in a single layer and bake for 25 to 28 minutes.

2. Meanwhile, add all of the pesto ingredients into a food processor and pulse until smooth. Transfer the mixture into a bowl and set aside.

3. For the zucchini mixture, in a large skill heat the oil on a medium heat. Add the garlic and Serrano pepper and sauté for about 1 minute. Add the zucchini, salt and black pepper and cook for 2 to 3 minutes. Add the pesto and gently stir to coat well. Cook for 1 minute. Transfer the zucchini mixture into a large serving bowl. Top with the meatballs and serve.

Zucchini with Turkey

The fresh zucchini, bell peppers and spices form a beautiful combination with the turkey in this dish. This is a super family friendly recipe that is ideal for dinner anytime of the week.

MAKES: 4 servings
PREPARATION TIME: 20 minutes
COOKING TIME: 20 minutes

2 tablespoons Extra Virgin Olive Oil

2 cups Grass-Fed boneless Turkey, cubed

Sea Salt, to taste

Freshly Ground Black Pepper, to taste

½ cup Yellow Onion, chopped

½ cup Green Bell Pepper, seeded and chopped

½ cup Red Bell Pepper, seeded and chopped

½ cup Yellow Bell Pepper, seeded and chopped

½ cup Orange Bell Pepper, seeded and chopped

2 Garlic Cloves, minced

1 Jalapeño Pepper, seeded and chopped

½ teaspoon Dried Oregano, crushed

¼ teaspoon Red Chili Powder

3 large Zucchinis, spiralized

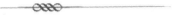

Directions

1. In a large skillet, heat 1 tablespoon of the oil on a medium heat. Add the turkey and sprinkle with salt and black pepper. Cook for 6 to 8 minutes, or until cooked. Transfer the turkey onto a plate. In the same skillet, heat the remaining oil. Add the onion and bell peppers and sauté for 5 to 7 minutes. Add the garlic, jalapeño pepper, oregano and red chili and sauté for 1 minute more.

2. Stir in the zucchini, salt and black pepper and cook for 3 to 4 minutes. Return the turkey to the pan before removing from the heat and serving hot.

Turkey & Mushroom Pasta

This recipe of zucchini noodles with ground turkey meat, mushroom and tomato sauce makes a surprisingly delicious meal for family and friends.

MAKES: 4 servings
PREPARATION TIME: 15 minutes
COOKING TIME: 35 minutes

2 tablespoons Extra Virgin Olive Oil

1 cup White Onion, chopped

1 pound Grass-Fed Lean Ground Turkey

2 Garlic Cloves, minced

1 cup Shiitake Mushrooms, sliced

4 cups Roma Tomatoes, chopped

Sea Salt, to taste

Freshly Ground Black Pepper, to taste

1 cup Homemade Chicken Broth

3 large Zucchinis, spiralized

½ cup Fresh Parsley, chopped

Directions

3. In a large skillet, heat 1 tablespoon of the oil on a medium heat. Sauté the onion for 4 to 5 minutes. Add the garlic and sauté for 1 minute before adding the mushrooms and cooking for 4 to 5 minutes. Add the turkey and cook for 5 to 6 minutes. Add the tomatoes, salt and black pepper and cook for 2 to 3 minutes whilst crushing the tomatoes with the back of a spoon. Add the broth and bring to a boil before reducing the heat and simmering for 10 to 15 minutes.
4. Meanwhile, in another skillet, heat the remaining oil on a medium heat. Add the zucchini, salt and black pepper and cook for 4 to 5 minutes. Transfer the zucchini onto a large serving plate. Top with the turkey gravy. Garnish with parsley and serve hot.

Spaghetti & Turkey Meatballs in Tomato Sauce

These zucchini noodles and turkey meatballs combine deliciously with the tomato sauce to make a great tasting and satisfying dinner that is easily prepared.

MAKES: 4 servings
PREPARATION TIME: 20 minutes
COOKING TIME: 45 minutes

For Meatballs:

1 pound Grass-Fed Lean Ground Turkey

2 Garlic Cloves, minced

¼ cup Parsley, freshly chopped

1 Organic Egg, beaten

2 tablespoons Blanched Almond Flour

2 tablespoons Coconut Aminos

Sea Salt, to taste

Freshly Ground Black Pepper, to taste

2 tablespoons Extra Virgin Olive Oil

For Tomato Sauce:

2 teaspoons Extra Virgin Olive Oil

¼ Yellow Onion, chopped

2-3 Garlic Cloves, minced

1 Jalapeño Pepper, seeded and chopped

1 tablespoon Rosemary, freshly chopped

½ teaspoon Red Pepper Flakes, crushed

3¼ cups Plum Tomatoes, finely chopped

¾ cup Homemade Chicken Broth

Sea Salt, to taste

Freshly Ground Black Pepper, to taste

For Zucchini:
1 tablespoon Extra Virgin Olive Oil

3 large Zucchinis, spiralized

Sea Salt, to taste

Freshly Ground Black Pepper, to taste

Directions

1. In a large bowl, combine together all of the meatball ingredients, except for the oil. Make your desired sized balls from the mixture. In a large skillet, heat the oil on a medium heat. Add the meatballs and cook for 2 minutes per side. Transfer the meatballs onto a plate and set aside.
2. In the same skillet, heat the oil for the sauce. Sauté

the onion for 4 to 5 minutes on a medium heat Sauté the garlic, jalapeño pepper, rosemary and red pepper flakes for 1 minute more. To the skillet add the tomatoes and broth, and bring to a boil before reducing the heat and simmering for 15 to 20 minutes. Remove the pan from the heat and let it cool slightly. Transfer the sauce mixture into a blender and pulse until smooth. Return the sauce into the skillet and bring to a gentle simmer on a medium heat. Reduce the heat to low and stir in the meatballs, salt and black pepper, and cook for 10 to 15 minutes.

3. Meanwhile, for the zucchini, heat the oil on a medium heat in another skillet. Add the zucchini, salt and black pepper and cook for 4 to 5 minutes. Transfer the zucchini onto a large serving plate. Top with the meatballs and sauce, and serve hot.

6

BEEF, PORK & LAMB RECIPES

Zucchini Beef Salad

This is a versatile, healthy and great tasting salad with a delicious burst of flavors. This salad is guaranteed to amuse family and friends.

MAKES: 4 servings
PREPARATION TIME: 15 minutes (plus time to marinate)
COOKING TIME: 8 minutes

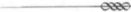

1 (1¼ pounds) Grass-Fed Flank Steak, trimmed

1 tablespoon Extra Virgin Olive Oil

Sea Salt, to taste

Freshly Ground Black Pepper, to taste

2 large Zucchinis, spiralized

1 Red Bell Pepper, seeded and thinly sliced

1 Orange Bell Pepper, seeded and thinly sliced

4 Radishes, julienned

2 cups Romaine Lettuce, torn

1 Ripe Avocado, peeled, pitted and chopped

For Dressing:
1 cup minced Cilantro

1 cup Parsley, freshly chopped

2 Garlic Cloves, minced

2 jalapeños, seeded and chopped

¼ cup Extra Virgin Olive Oil

¼ cup Fresh Lemon juice

Sea Salt, to taste

Freshly Ground Black Pepper, to taste

Directions

1. Preheat the grill to high and grease the grill grate. Drizzle the steak with the oil and sprinkle with the salt and black pepper. Set aside for 10 to 15 minutes before cooking the steak for about 4 minutes per

side. Transfer the steak onto a plate and set aside for 5 minutes. With a sharp knife, cut the steak into thin slices diagonally across the grain. Transfer the steak into a large serving bowl. Add the remaining salad ingredients to the bowl, except for the avocado, and mix.

2. In a food processor, add all of the dressing ingredients and pulse until smooth. Combine the dressing with the salad and toss to coat well. Top with the avocado and serve immediately.

Zucchini Lamb Chops Salad

This is a fantastic salad with fresh zucchini noodles and roasted lamb chops. This wonderful salad makes a light yet delicious weeknight meal.

MAKES: 4 servings
PREPARATION TIME: 20 minutes (plus time to marinate)
COOKING TIME: 16 minutes

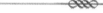

2 tablespoons Extra Virgin Olive Oil

1 tablespoon Fresh Rosemary, minced

2-3 Garlic Cloves, minced

Sea Salt, to taste

Freshly Ground Black Pepper, to taste

4 Grass-Fed Lamb Loin Chops

3 large Zucchinis, spiralized

1 tablespoon Fresh Lemon juice

2 tablespoons Scallion Leaves, freshly chopped

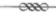

Directions

1. Preheat the oven to 400 degrees F. In a bowl, mix together 1 tablespoon of oil, rosemary, garlic, salt

111

and black pepper. Add the chops and generously coat with the marinade. Cover and refrigerate to marinate for 1 to 2 hours. In an ovenproof skillet, heat the remaining oil on a high heat. Add the chops and cook for about 6 minutes, turning once after 3 minutes. Place the skillet into the oven and roast for about 10 minutes.

2. Place the zucchini into a large serving bowl, sprinkle with salt and black pepper, and drizzle with the lemon juice. Gently toss to coat the zucchini before topping with the chops. Garnish with the scallion and serve.

Zucchini Steak Soup

This is an excellent recipe for a warm and comforting soup. This dish is a wonderful combination of beef and zucchini noodle with mushrooms and spinach.

MAKES: 2 servings
PREPARATION TIME: 20 minutes
COOKING TIME: 30 minutes

1½ tablespoons Extra Virgin Olive Oil

½ pound Grass-Fed, cubed, New York Strip Steak

Sea Salt, to taste

Freshly Ground Black Pepper, to taste

1 small Onion, chopped

3-4 Garlic Cloves, minced

1 cup Shiitake Mushrooms, chopped

1 cup Fresh Spinach, torn

3 cups Homemade Beef Broth

2 tablespoons Coconut Aminos

2 medium Zucchinis, spiralized

½ cup Scallions, chopped

Directions

1. In a large soup pan, heat 1 tablespoon of the oil on a medium heat. Add the beef and sprinkle with the salt and black pepper. Cook for 4 to 5 minutes, or until golden brown on all sides. Transfer the beef into a bowl. In the same pan, heat the remaining oil on a medium heat. Sauté the onion and for 4 to 5 minutes before adding and sautéing the garlic for 1 minute. Add the mushrooms and cook for 3 to 4 minutes. Add the spinach and cook for a further 2 to 3 minutes.

2. Add the broth and coconut aminos to the pan and bring to a boil before reducing the heat and simmering for about 5 minutes. Stir in the beef and simmer for a further 2 to 3 minutes. Stir in the zucchini, scallions, salt and black pepper and simmer for 2 to 3 minutes more. Remove the pan from the heat and serve hot.

Zucchini Ground Beef Soup

This is a satisfying, very easy and tasty zucchini, tomato and ground beef soup. This soup will be a great hit to serve anytime of the year.

MAKES: 4 servings
PREPARATION TIME: 15 minutes
COOKING TIME: 40 minutes

½ tablespoon Extra Virgin Olive Oil

¼ cup White Onion, chopped

2 Celery Stalks, chopped

½ cup Green Bell Pepper, seeded and chopped

½ pound Grass-Fed Ground Beef

3 cups Fresh Tomatoes, finely chopped

4 cups Homemade Beef Broth

1 tablespoon Fresh Thyme, minced

3 medium Zucchinis, spiralized

Sea Salt, to taste

Freshly Ground Black Pepper, to taste

1 tablespoon Fresh Lemon juice

½ cup Scallions, chopped (plus additional scallions for garnishing)

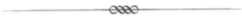

Directions

1. In a large soup pan, heat the oil on a medium heat. Sauté the onion, celery and bell pepper for 4 to 5 minutes. Add the beef and cook for 4 to 5 minutes. Add the tomatoes and cook for a further 1 to 2 minutes. Add the broth and thyme and bring to a boil before reducing the heat, covering, and simmering for 20 to 25 minutes.
2. Stir in the zucchini, scallions, salt and black pepper, and simmer for 2 to 3 minutes more. Stir in lemon juice and remove from the heat. Garnish with additional scallions and serve hot.

Spicy Zucchini Lamb Soup

This soup is a wonderfully delicious dish with a nice spicy kick. It is nourishing, filling and healthy.

MAKES: 4 servings
PREPARATION TIME: 15 minutes
COOKING TIME: 1 hour 50 minutes

---

1 tablespoon Extra Virgin Olive Oil

1 medium Yellow Onion, chopped

2 large Grass-Fed Lamb Shanks

2 Celery Stalks, chopped

2 small Carrots, peeled and chopped

2 Garlic Cloves, minced

1 teaspoon Fresh Ginger, minced

½ teaspoon Dried Oregano, crushed

½ teaspoon Dried Thyme, crushed

1 teaspoon Ground Cilantro

1½ teaspoons Ground Cumin

½ teaspoon Cayenne Pepper

2 cups Tomatoes, chopped

6 cups Homemade Chicken Broth

3 medium Zucchinis, spiralized

Sea Salt, to taste

Freshly Ground Black Pepper, to taste

½ cup Fresh Parsley, chopped

Directions

1. In a large soup pan, heat the oil on a medium heat. Add the shanks and cook for 6 to 8 minutes, until browned on all sides. Transfer the shanks into a bowl and set aside. In the same pan, sauté the onion, celery and carrot for 4 to 5 minutes. Add the garlic, ginger, herbs and spices and sauté for a further minute. Add the tomatoes and cook for 1 to 2 minutes more. Add the cooked shanks and broth to the pan and bring to a boil before reducing the heat and simmering, partially covered, for about 1½ hours.

2. Remove the shanks from the soup and shred the meat. Return the shredded meat to the pan with the zucchini, salt and black pepper, and simmer for 3 to 4 minutes. Garnish with parsley and serve hot.

Stir Fried Zucchini & Beef

This quick and easy stir fry recipe combines beef and zucchini for a dish packed with nutrients and flavor.

MAKES: 2 servings
PREPARATION TIME: 10 minutes
COOKING TIME: 13 minutes

1½ tablespoons Olive Oil, Extra Virgin

½ pound Grass-Fed boneless Fillet, sliced thinly

Sea Salt, to taste

Freshly Ground Black Pepper, to taste

1 small Onion, chopped

1 Garlic Clove, minced

½ teaspoon Fresh Ginger, minced

1 tablespoon Coconut Aminos

2 large Zucchinis, spiralized

1 tablespoon Basil Leaves, freshly chopped

1 teaspoon Black Sesame Seeds

Directions

1. Heat the oil on a medium-high heat in a skillet. Add the beef and sprinkle with salt and black pepper before stir frying for 2 to 3 minutes. Transfer the beef onto a plate to set aside. In the same skillet, add the onion on a medium heat and sauté for 4 to 5 minutes. Add the garlic and ginger and sauté for 1 minute more. Stir in the coconut aminos and cook for a further minute.
2. Stir in the zucchini, salt and black pepper and stir fry for 2 minutes. Add the beef and cook for 1 to 2 minutes more. Stir in basil leaves and remove from heat. Garnish with the sesame seeds and serve.

Sautéed Zucchini with Grilled Beef

This is a great recipe to incorporate zucchini and beef together. This super easy meal will be a hit for midweek quick dinners.

MAKES: 4 servings
PREPARATION TIME: 10 minutes (plus time to marinate)
COOKING TIME: 10 minutes

For Beef:

2 Beets, trimmed

1 tablespoon Extra Virgin Olive Oil

2 Garlic Cloves, minced

2 teaspoons Fresh Thyme, minced

2 teaspoons Fresh Oregano, minced

1 teaspoon Lime Zest, freshly grated

Sea Salt, to taste

Freshly Ground Black Pepper, to taste

1½ pounds Grass-Fed Beef Tri-Tip, cut into 4 steaks lengthwise

For Zucchini:
1 tablespoon Extra Virgin Olive Oil

1 Garlic Clove, minced

¼ teaspoon Red Pepper Flakes, crushed

3 medium Zucchinis, spiralized

Sea Salt, to taste

Freshly Ground Black Pepper, to taste

1 tablespoon Fresh Lime Juice

Directions

1. In a large bowl, mix together all of the beef ingredients, except for the steak. Add the steaks and generously coat with the beef ingredients mixture. Set aside for at least 30 minutes to marinate. Preheat the grill to medium-high and grease the grill grate. Cook the steaks for about 5 minutes per side before transferring to a bowl.
2. Meanwhile, for the zucchini, in a skillet heat the oil on a medium heat and sauté the garlic and red pepper flakes for about 1 minute. Add the zucchini, salt and black pepper and cook for 3 to 4 minutes. Stir in the lime juice and remove from the heat before transferring the zucchini onto a serving plate, topping with the steak and serving.

Zucchini with Ground Beef

This recipe is for a healthy and delicious skillet dinner using zucchini, cherry tomatoes and ground beef. This dish will quickly become a staple part of your repertoire.

MAKES: 4 servings
PREPARATION TIME: 10 minutes
COOKING TIME: 15 minutes

1 tablespoon Extra Virgin Olive Oil

1 medium Onion, chopped

2 Garlic Cloves, minced

1 pound Grass-Fed Lean Ground Beef

¼ cup Homemade Beef Broth

1 cup Cherry Tomatoes, halved

3 medium Zucchinis, spiralized

Sea Salt, to taste

Freshly Ground Black Pepper, to taste

3 tablespoons Basil, freshly chopped

Directions

1. In a large skillet, heat the oil on a medium heat and sauté the onion and garlic for about 1 minute. Add the beef and cook, stirring, for 4 to 5 minutes. Add the tomatoes and broth, and cook for 4 to 5 minutes.
2. Stir in the zucchini, salt and black pepper and cook for 3 to 4 minutes. Stir in the basil and remove from heat before serving hot.

Zoodles & Meatballs

This is a nice and tasty addition to your main entrée meals. Your entire family, especially your kids, will love to enjoy this meal.

MAKES: 4 servings
PREPARATION TIME: 20 minutes
COOKING TIME: 40 minutes

For Meatballs:

1½ pounds Grass-Fed Lean Ground Beef

3 tablespoons Parsley, freshly chopped

¼ cup Onion, chopped

2 Garlic Cloves, minced

1 large Organic Egg, beaten

2 tablespoons Flax Meal

¼ teaspoon Red Pepper Flakes, crushed

Sea Salt, to taste

Freshly Ground Black Pepper, to taste

For Zucchini:

1 tablespoon Extra Virgin Olive Oil

4-5 Garlic Cloves, minced

1 Cup Portobello Mushrooms, chopped

2 medium Zucchinis, spiralized

1 cup Black Olives, pitted and sliced

Sea Salt, to taste

Freshly Ground Black Pepper, to taste

½ cup Parsley, freshly chopped

Directions

1. Preheat the oven to 375 degrees F and line a baking dish with parchment paper. For the meatballs, mix together all of the meatball ingredients in a bowl. Make your desired sized balls from the mixture and arrange the balls in the prepared baking dish in a single layer. Cover with foil and bake for about 30 minutes. Remove the foil and bake for 10 minutes more.
2. Meanwhile, for the zucchini, heat the oil on a medium heat in a large skillet. Sauté the garlic for about 1 minute. Add the mushrooms and sauté for 4 to 5 minutes. Add the zucchini, olives, salt and black pepper and cook for 3 to 4 minutes. Stir in the parsley and remove from heat. Transfer the zucchini mixture onto a serving plate. Top with the meatballs and serve.

Zucchini & Beef Stew

This recipe wonderfully combines the warmth of the beef with zucchini noodle. The carrots, celery and spices in this dish really enhanced the flavor of the stew.

MAKES: 4 servings
PREPARATION TIME: 20 minutes
COOKING TIME: 1 hour 30 minutes

½ tablespoon Extra Virgin Olive Oil

1 pound Grass-Fed Beef Stew, cubed

Sea Salt, to taste

Freshly Ground Black Pepper, to taste

1 medium Onion, chopped

4 Celery Stalks, chopped

2 large Carrots, peeled and chopped

2 Garlic Cloves, minced

1 Serrano pepper, chopped

2 Bay leaves

1 teaspoon Dried Thyme, crushed

1 teaspoon Ground Cilantro

2 teaspoons Ground Cumin

½ teaspoon Cayenne Pepper

2 cups Tomatoes, finely chopped

5 cups Homemade Chicken Broth

2 tablespoons Coconut Aminos

2 large Zucchinis, spiralized

2 Yellow Squash, spiralized

½ cup fresh Basil, chopped

Directions

1. In a large pan, heat the oil on a medium heat. Add the beef and cook for 4 to 5 minutes, until browned on all sides. Transfer the beef into a bowl. In the same pan, add the onion, celery and carrot and sauté for 5 to 6 minutes. Add the garlic, Serrano pepper, bay leaves, thyme and spices and sauté for 1 minute more. Add the tomatoes to the pan and cook for 2 to 3 minutes. Add the beef, broth and coconut aminos and bring to a boil before reducing the heat and simmering, partially covered, for about 40 minutes. Uncover and simmer for a further 25 to 30 minutes.
2. Stir in the zucchini, squash, salt and black pepper and cook for 4 to 5 minutes. Garnish with the basil and serve.

Zucchini & Lamb Stew

This recipe combines zucchini and lamb to be cooked together for an irresistibly delicious one skillet entrée. This truly is a fantastic way to enjoy zucchini with lamb!

MAKES: 4 servings
PREPARATION TIME: 15 minutes
COOKING TIME: 1 hour 35 minutes

---

1 tablespoon Extra Virgin Olive Oil

1 pound Grass-Fed boneless, trimmed and cubed Lamb Leg

1 cup White Onion, chopped

1½ cups Carrots, peeled and thinly sliced

½ teaspoon Ground Ginger

3½ cups Homemade Chicken Broth

2 large Zucchinis, spiralized

Sea Salt, to taste

Freshly Ground Black Pepper, to taste

1 tablespoon Fresh Lime juice

½ cup Fresh Scallions, chopped

Directions

1. In a large pan, heat the oil on a medium-high heat. Add the lamb and cook for about 5 minutes, until browned on all sides. Transfer the lamb into a bowl. In the same pan, sauté the onion and carrot for 4 to 5 minutes. Add the cooked lamb, ginger and broth and bring to a boil before reducing the heat and simmering, covered, for about 1 hour and 20 minutes.
2. Stir in the zucchini, salt and black pepper and cook for 4 to 5 minutes. Add the lime juice, stir, and remove the pan from the heat before garnishing with the scallions and serving.

Zucchini Olives & Ground Lamb

This is a dish with a touch of gourmet and elegance! In this dish the ground lamb provides a lovely richness to the zucchini and olives.

MAKES: 4 servings
PREPARATION TIME: 15 minutes
COOKING TIME: 20 minutes

2 Garlic Cloves, minced

1 teaspoon Extra Virgin Olive Oil

1 pound Grass-Fed Lean Ground Lamb

½ teaspoon Red Pepper Flakes, crushed

½ cup Fresh Tomatoes, finely chopped

2 large Zucchinis, spiralized

1 cup Black Olives, pitted and sliced

Sea Salt, to taste

Freshly Ground Black Pepper, to taste

¼ cup Scallions, chopped

Directions

1. In a large skillet, heat the oil on a medium-high heat and sauté the garlic for about 1 minute. Add the lamb and sprinkle with the red pepper flakes. Cook, stirring occasionally, for 8 to 10 minutes. Add the tomatoes to the skillet and cook for 3 to 4 minutes.
2. Stir in the zucchini, olives, salt and black pepper, and cook for 4 to 5 minutes. Top with the scallions and serve.

Spicy Zucchini with Ground Lamb

This is one of the best dishes for spice lovers! The combination of spices, herbs and lemon juice really brightens the flavors of the zucchini and lamb.

MAKES: 4 servings
PREPARATION TIME: 15 minutes
COOKING TIME: 25 minutes

2 tablespoons Coconut Oil, Extra Virgin

1 medium Onion, chopped

2 Garlic Cloves, minced

1 teaspoon Fresh Ginger, minced

1 Jalapeño Pepper, seeded and chopped

½ teaspoon Dried Rosemary, crushed

½ teaspoon Dried Thyme, crushed

½ teaspoon Ground Cilantro

1 teaspoon Ground Cumin

¼ teaspoon Ground Turmeric

½ teaspoon Cayenne Pepper

1 pound Grass-Fed Lean Ground Lamb

3 large Zucchinis, spiralized

Sea Salt, to taste

Freshly Ground Black Pepper, to taste

2 tablespoons Fresh Lime juice

¼ cup minced Cilantro Leaves

Directions

1. In a large skillet, heat the oil on a medium heat. Sauté the onion for 4 to 5 minutes. Add the garlic, ginger, jalapeño pepper, herbs and spices and sauté for a further minute. Add the lamb and cook for 10 to 12 minutes while stirring occasionally.
2. Stir in the zucchini, salt and black pepper and cook for 4 to 5 minutes. Stir in the lime juice and cilantro and cook for 1 to 2 minutes more before serving hot.

Green Zucchini & Meatballs

This is a fantastic and healthy recipe when planning a meal for a family gathering.

MAKES: 4 servings
PREPARATION TIME: 15 minutes
COOKING TIME: 8 minutes

For Meatballs:

1 pound Grass-Fed Lean Ground Lamb

1 Organic Egg, beaten

2 Garlic Cloves, minced

1 medium White Onion, finely chopped

¼ teaspoon Ground Cumin

Sea Salt, to taste

Freshly Ground Black Pepper, to taste

1 tablespoon Extra Virgin Olive Oil

For Zucchini:

1 tablespoon Extra Virgin Olive Oil

2 Garlic Cloves, minced

4 medium Zucchinis, spiralized

Sea Salt, to taste

Freshly Ground Black Pepper, to taste

For Sauce:

1 cup Fresh Parsley Leaves

1 cup Fresh Mint Leaves

2 Garlic Cloves, minced

¼ cup Extra Virgin Olive Oil

1 tablespoon Fresh Lime juice

Pinch of Cayenne Pepper

Sea Salt, to taste

Freshly Ground Black Pepper, to taste

Directions

1. Preheat the grill to high and grease the grill grate. In a bowl, mix together all of the meatball ingredients, except for the oil. Make your desired sized balls from the mixture. Coat the balls with the oil and grill the balls for about 8 minutes, turning once after 4 minutes. Transfer the balls into a bowl.
2. Meanwhile, for the zucchini, heat the oil on a medium heat in a skillet. Sauté the garlic for about 1 minute. Add the zucchini, salt and black pepper and cook for about 4 to 5 minutes. Transfer the zucchini onto a large serving plate.
3. Add all of the sauce ingredients into a food

processor and pulse until smooth. Pour the sauce over the zucchini and toss to coat. Top with the grilled meatballs and serve.

Zucchini with Pork Chops

This recipe makes a comforting and tasty dish. This meal is prepared with simple ingredients but is very rich in flavors.

MAKES: 4 servings
PREPARATION TIME: 15 minutes
COOKING TIME: 14 minutes

For Pork Chops:

2 tablespoons Coconut Oil, Extra Virgin

4 boneless Pork Chops

¼ teaspoon Cayenne Pepper

Sea Salt, to taste

Freshly Ground Black Pepper, to taste

For Zucchini:

1 tablespoon Coconut Oil, Extra Virgin

2 Garlic Cloves, minced

4 medium Zucchinis, spiralized

Sea Salt, to taste

Freshly Ground Black Pepper, to taste

1 teaspoon Lemon Zest, freshly grated

Directions

1. Preheat the oven to 400 degrees F. Heat the oil in a large oven proof skillet on a medium-high heat. Add the chops and sprinkle with the cayenne pepper, salt and black pepper, and sear for about 6 minutes, turning once after 3 minutes. Transfer the skillet into the oven and roast the chops until cooked, for about 8 minutes.

2. Meanwhile, for the zucchini, heat the oil on medium heat in another skillet. Sauté the garlic for about 1 minute before adding the zucchini, salt and black pepper and cooking for 4 to 5 minutes. Transfer the zucchini onto a large serving plate. Top with the chops, garnish with the lemon zest and serve.

Garlicky Zucchini & Pork

This is a gorgeous and easy to cook recipe for the whole family. The combination of ingredients gives an amazingly delicious flavor to this dish.

MAKES: 4 servings
PREPARATION TIME: 15 minutes
COOKING TIME: 15 minutes

---

1 tablespoon Coconut Oil, Extra Virgin

2-3 Garlic Cloves, minced

1 pound Lean Ground Pork

1 Serrano Pepper, seeded and chopped

1 tablespoon fresh Ginger, grated

1 tablespoon fresh Thyme, chopped

1 tablespoon Coconut Vinegar

2 tablespoons Coconut Aminos

2 small Carrots, peeled and spiralized

4 medium Zucchinis, spiralized

1 cup Black Olives, pitted and chopped

Sea Salt, to taste

Freshly Ground Black Pepper, to taste

¼ cup Parsley, freshly chopped

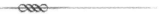

Directions

1. In a large skillet, heat the oil on a medium-high heat. Sauté the garlic for about 1 minute. Add the pork and cook for 5 to 6 minutes. Add the Serrano pepper, ginger and thyme and cook for 1 minute more. Add the vinegar and coconut aminos and cook for a further 2 minutes.

2. Stir in the carrots and cook for about 2 minutes. Stir in the zucchini, olives, salt and black pepper and cook for 2 to 3 minutes. Garnish with the parsley and serve hot.

7

FISH & SEAFOOD RECIPES

Zucchini & Salmon Salad

This is a fantastic recipe for spiralized zucchini, tomatoes and olives with grilled salmon. The dressing with this dish adds a refreshingly delicious touch to this salad.

MAKES: 4 servings
PREPARATION TIME: 20 minutes
COOKING TIME: 8 minutes

For Salmon:

4 (4-ounce) Salmon Fillets

1 tablespoon Extra Virgin Olive Oil

Sea Salt, to taste

Freshly Ground Black Pepper, to taste

For Salad:

2 small Zucchinis, spiralized

1 cup Cherry Tomatoes, halved

¼ cup Black Olives, pitted and sliced

3 tablespoons Extra Virgin Olive Oil

3 tablespoon Fresh Lime juice

2 teaspoons Lime Zest, freshly grated

¼ cup Fresh Cilantro Leaves, minced

Sea Salt, to taste

Freshly Ground Black Pepper, to taste

¼ cup Walnuts, toasted and chopped

Directions

1. Preheat the grill to high and grease the grill grate. Place the salmon fillets in a dish, drizzle with the oil and sprinkle with the salt and black pepper. Grill the salmon for about 4 minutes per side. Remove from the grill and transfer into a bowl.
2. In a large serving bowl, mix together the zucchini, tomatoes and olives. In another small bowl, beat together the oil, lime juice, zest, cilantro, salt and black pepper. Combine the dressing with the salad

and mix thoroughly. Top with the salmon and walnuts, and serve immediately.

Zucchini & Shrimp Salad

This is a great tasting, healthy and fresh salad which has marvelous flavors.

MAKES: 2 servings
PREPARATION TIME: 15 minutes
COOKING TIME: 5 minutes

For Salad:

1 tablespoon Extra Virgin Olive Oil

2 Garlic Cloves, minced

1 teaspoon Fresh Ginger, minced

½ pound Shrimp, peeled and deveined

Sea Salt, to taste

Freshly Ground Black Pepper, to taste

2 medium Zucchinis, spiralized

3 cups mixed Fresh Baby Greens

1 small Avocado, peeled, pitted and chopped

For Dressing:

1 tablespoon Extra Virgin Olive Oil

1 tablespoon Fresh Lemon juice

1 tablespoon Coconut Aminos

½ teaspoon Raw Honey

Pinch of Red Pepper Flakes, crushed

Sea Salt, to taste

Freshly Ground Black Pepper, to taste

Directions

1. In a skillet, heat the oil on a medium heat. Sauté the garlic and ginger for about 1 minute. Add the shrimp and sprinkle with salt and black pepper. Cook for about 4 minutes, turning once after 2 minutes. Transfer the shrimp into a large serving bowl. Add the zucchini and greens to the shrimp.
2. In another bowl, beat together all of the dressing ingredients before pouring the dressing over the salad and gently tossing to coat. Garnish with the avocado and serve immediately.

Lemony Zucchini & Herring Soup

This soup is filled with the healthy flavors of herring fish, ginger, lemon and zucchini. The slight tangy flavor in this dish nicely compliments its earthy taste.

MAKES: 2 servings
PREPARATION TIME: 15 minutes
COOKING TIME: 10 minutes

1 tablespoon Extra Virgin Olive Oil

1 teaspoon Fresh Ginger, finely grated

2 (3-ounce) Herring Fillets

Sea Salt, to taste

Freshly Ground Black Pepper, to taste

2 cups Homemade Vegetable Broth

½ Jalapeño Pepper, seeded and minced

2 medium Zucchinis, spiralized

1 tablespoon Fresh Lemon juice

¼ cup Scallion, chopped

¼ teaspoon Lemon Zest, freshly grated

Directions

1. In a large skillet, heat the oil on a medium-high heat. Sauté the ginger for about 1 minute. Add the herring and sprinkle with salt and black pepper. Cook for about 8 minutes, turning once after 4 minutes.
2. Meanwhile, in a soup pan add the broth and bring to a boil on a high heat. Reduce the heat to medium and stir in the jalapeño pepper and zucchini. Cook for about 2 to 3 minutes. Stir in the cooked herring, lemon juice, salt and black pepper and remove from the heat.
3. Top with the scallions and lemon zest before serving hot.

Zoodles & Salmon Soup

This hearty yet light soup has many delicious flavors, and it is sure to warm you up in the cold winter weather.

MAKES: 2 servings
PREPARATION TIME: 15 minutes
COOKING TIME: 10 minutes

2 (3-ounce) Salmon Fillets

Sea Salt, to taste

Freshly Ground Black Pepper, to taste

1 tablespoon Extra Virgin Olive Oil

2 Garlic Cloves, minced

1 teaspoon Fresh Ginger, minced

1½ cups Fresh Spinach, torn

2 cups Homemade Vegetable Broth

2 tablespoons Coconut Aminos

2 medium Zucchinis, spiralized

¼ cup Scallions, chopped

Directions

1. Set a steamer basket over a pan of boiling water. Add the salmon fillets and sprinkle with salt and black pepper. Cover and steam for 5 to 6 minutes.
2. Meanwhile, in a large skillet heat the oil on a medium heat. Sauté the garlic and ginger for about 1 minute. Add the spinach and cook for 2 to 3 minutes. Add the broth and coconut aminos and bring to a boil. Stir in the zucchini, salt and black pepper and cook for 4 to 5 minutes. Sir in the salmon and scallions and remove from the heat before serving hot.

Spicy Zucchini & Herring Stew

*This is an awesome and healthy stew with a tangy and spicy kick!
This stew will be a great hit for the cold winter season.*

MAKES: 4 servings
PREPARATION TIME: 15 minutes
COOKING TIME: 25 minutes

———————⟨∞⟩———————

1 tablespoon Extra Virgin Olive Oil

1 Yellow Onion, chopped

3-4 Garlic Cloves, minced

½ teaspoon Dried Oregano, crushed

1 teaspoon Ground Cumin

½ teaspoon Ground Cilantro

½ teaspoon Cayenne Pepper

4 cups Fresh Tomatoes, finely chopped

¼ cup Black Olives, pitted and sliced

1 tablespoon Capers

2 cups Homemade Fish Broth

1 pound (453g) Herring, cubed

1 pound (453g) Zucchini, spiralized

Sea Salt, to taste

Freshly Ground Black Pepper, to taste

2 tablespoons Fresh Lemon juice

¼ cup Fresh Cilantro Leaves, minced

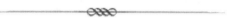

Directions

1. In a large pan, heat the oil on a medium heat. Sauté the onion for 4 to 5 minutes. Add the garlic, herbs and spices and sauté for about 1 minute. Add the tomatoes and cook for 1 to 2 minutes. Add the olives, capers and broth and bring to a boil. Reduce the heat to medium-low and simmer for about 10 minutes.

2. Stir in the fish and cook for a further 3 to 4 minutes. Stir in the zucchini, salt and black pepper and cook for 2 to 3 minutes more. Stir in the lemon juice and cilantro and immediately remove from the heat before serving hot.

Baked Zucchini Mushrooms & Cod

This recipe makes a surprisingly filling, light and delicious meal for the whole family. The cod fish holds together nicely when baked with zucchini and mushrooms.

MAKES: 4 servings
PREPARATION TIME: 15 minutes
COOKING TIME: 30 minutes

2 tablespoons Extra Virgin Olive Oil

1 medium White onion

½ teaspoon Dried Rosemary, crushed

2 cups Portabella Mushrooms, sliced

2 Large Zucchinis, spiralized

Sea Salt, to taste

Freshly Ground Black Pepper, to taste

4 (4-ounce) Cod Fillets

Directions

1. Preheat the oven to 450 degrees F and grease a

baking dish.

2. In a large skillet, heat the oil on a medium heat. Sauté the onion for 2 to 3 minutes. Add the rosemary and mushrooms and sauté for 3 to 4 minute. Add the zucchini, salt and black pepper and sauté for a further 3 minutes.

3. Sprinkle the fish fillets with salt and black pepper on both sides. Arrange the fish fillets in the prepared baking dish in a single layer. Top with the zucchini mixture and cover the baking dish with foil. Bake for 15 to 20 minutes, or until cooked.

Zucchini Baked Salmon Combo

This is a delicious dish which is packed with a hearty amount of healthy nutrients. This dish is guaranteed to become a favorite meal for your family.

MAKES: 2 servings
PREPARATION TIME: 15 minutes (plus time to marinate)
COOKING TIME: 15 minutes

2 tablespoons Extra Virgin Olive Oil

2 tablespoons Coconut Aminos

Sea Salt, to taste

Freshly Ground Black Pepper, to taste

1 (6-ounce) Salmon Fillet, cubed

2 Garlic Cloves, minced

½ teaspoon Fresh Ginger, minced

1 cup Oyster Mushrooms, stemmed

1 Carrot, peeled and spiralized

2 medium Zucchinis, spiralized

Directions

4. Preheat the oven to 400 degrees F and line a baking dish with parchment paper. In a medium bowl, mix together 1 tablespoon of oil, the coconut aminos, salt and black pepper. Add the salmon and toss to coat well. Set aside for at least 10 minutes to marinate. Transfer the salmon mixture into the prepared baking dish and bake for 10 to 15 minutes until cooked.

5. Meanwhile, in a large skillet heat the remaining oil on a medium heat. Sauté the garlic and ginger for about 1 minute. Add the mushrooms and cook for 4 to 5 minutes. Add the carrot and cook for 2 minutes more. Add the zucchini, salt and black pepper and cook for a further 3 minutes.

6. Place the zucchini mixture onto a serving plate, top with the salmon and serve hot.

Sautéed Zucchini & Shrimp

This is a filing and delicious meal which can be prepared very quickly. The combination of fresh lime juice and garlic compliments the shrimp and zucchini perfectly.

MAKES: 2 servings
PREPARATION TIME: 10 minutes
COOKING TIME: 10 minutes

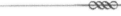

1½ tablespoons Coconut Oil, Extra Virgin

2 Garlic Cloves, minced

¼ cup Shallots, minced

Pinch of Red Pepper Flakes, crushed

1 pound Shrimp, peeled and deveined

3 tablespoons Fresh Lime juice

Sea Salt, to taste

Freshly Ground Black Pepper, to taste

3 medium Zucchinis, spiralized

2 tablespoons minced Cilantro Leaves

1 teaspoon Lime Zest, freshly grated

Directions

1. In a skillet, heat 1 tablespoon of oil on a medium heat. Sauté the garlic for about 1 minute. Add the shallot and red pepper flakes and sauté for about 1 minute. Add the shrimp and sprinkle with salt and black pepper. Cook for about 4 minutes, turning once after 2 minutes. Stir in the lime juice and immediately transfer the shrimp into a bowl.

2. In the same skillet, heat the remaining oil on a medium heat. Add the zucchini and sauté for 2 to 3 minutes. Stir in the shrimp and mix. Remove from the heat and transfer onto serving plates. Garnish with the cilantro and lime zest, and serve hot.

Stir Fried Zucchini & Shrimp

This dish is one of the healthiest and most delightful meals for all. The zucchini and asparagus compliment nicely with the shrimp in this dish.

MAKES: 4 servings
PREPARATION TIME: 15 minutes
COOKING TIME: 8 minutes

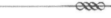

2 tablespoons Extra Virgin Olive Oil

2 Garlic Cloves, minced

1 cup Asparagus, trimmed and cut into 1-inch pieces

4 medium Zucchinis, spiralized

1 teaspoon Coconut Aminos

1 pound Shrimp, peeled and deveined

Sea Salt, to taste

Freshly Ground Black Pepper, to taste

3 tablespoons Fresh Parsley, chopped

1 tablespoon Black Sesame Seeds

Directions

1. In a skillet, heat the oil on a medium heat. Sauté the garlic for about 1 minute. Add the asparagus and zucchini and sauté for 2 to 3 minutes.
2. Add the coconut aminos, shrimp, salt and black pepper, and cook for about 4 minutes. Stir in the parsley and immediately remove from the heat. Garnish with the sesame seeds and serve hot.

Squash Noodles with Grilled Shrimp

This is a tasty and hearty dish of shrimp paired with zucchini and yellow squash. This dish not only tastes great, it is also prepared without spending much time in the kitchen.

MAKES: 4 servings
PREPARATION TIME: 10 minutes (plus time to marinate)
COOKING TIME: 10 minutes

For Shrimp:

2 Garlic Cloves, minced

1 teaspoon Fresh Rosemary, minced

1 teaspoon Fresh Oregano, minced

2 teaspoons Lemon Zest, freshly grated

2 tablespoons Extra Virgin Olive Oil

1 tablespoon Fresh Lemon juice

Sea Salt, to taste

Freshly Ground Black Pepper, to taste

1 pound Shrimp, peeled and deveined

For Vegetables:

1 tablespoon Extra Virgin Olive Oil

1 Garlic Clove, minced

2 medium Zucchinis, spiralized

2 medium Yellow Squash, spiralized

Sea Salt, to taste

Freshly Ground Black Pepper, to taste

½ tablespoon Fresh Lemon juice

Directions

1. For the shrimp, in a large bowl mix together all of the ingredients, except for the shrimp. Add the shrimp and generously coat with the marinade before covering and refrigerating for 2 to 3 hours. Remove the shrimp from the refrigerator and set aside at room temperature for 20 to 30 minutes. Preheat the grill to medium-high and grease the grill grate. Cook the shrimp for about 2 minutes per side. Transfer the shrimp into a bowl and cover loosely with foil to keep them warm.

2. In a skillet, heat the oil on a medium heat. Sauté the garlic for about 1 minute. Add the zucchini and squash and sauté for 4 to 5 minutes. Stir in the lemon juice and immediately remove from the heat. Adjust the taste with the salt and black pepper, if required. Transfer the zucchini mixture onto a serving plate, top with the shrimp and serve.

Zucchini & Broccoli Shrimp

This is an easy, rich and aromatic meal. This skillet meal is packed with the healthy nutrients of shrimp, zucchini and broccoli.

MAKES: 2 servings
PREPARATION TIME: 20 minutes
COOKING TIME: 15 minutes

¼ cup Coconut Aminos

1 tablespoon Fresh Lime juice

2 teaspoons Raw Honey

1 small Onion, chopped

2 tablespoons Extra Virgin Olive Oil

1 cup Broccoli Florets

1 teaspoon Fresh Ginger, minced

2 Garlic Cloves, minced

1 large Red Bell Pepper, seeded and sliced thinly

Sea Salt, to taste

Freshly Ground Black Pepper, to taste

½ pound Shrimp, peeled and deveined

2 large Zucchinis, spiralized

1 teaspoon Black Sesame Seeds

Directions

1. In a bowl, mix together the coconut aminos, lime juice and honey and set aside. In a skillet, heat 1 tablespoon of oil on a medium heat. Sauté the onion for 3 to 4 minutes. Add the broccoli and cook for 3 to 4 minutes. Add the bell pepper, ginger and garlic and sauté for about 2 minutes. Stir in the salt and black pepper.
2. Add the shrimp and cook for about 2 minutes. Add the honey mixture and zucchini and cook for a further 2 to 3 minutes. Transfer the mixture into a serving bowl. Top with the sesame seeds and serve.

Zucchini Shrimp & Clams

This is a wonderfully delicious dish of zucchini pasta with shrimp and clams. This dish will be a hit with the whole family at dinner time.

MAKES: 4 servings
PREPARATION TIME: 15 minutes
COOKING TIME: 10 minutes

2 tablespoons Extra Virgin Olive Oil

2-3 Garlic Cloves, minced

12 Clams, scrubbed

¼ cup Homemade Fish Broth

1 pound Shrimp, peeled and deveined

Sea Salt, to taste

Freshly Ground Black Pepper, to taste

1 tablespoon Fresh Lime juice

4 large Zucchinis, spiralized

3 tablespoons Parsleyfreshly chopped

Directions

1. In a skillet, heat the oil on a medium heat. Sauté the garlic for about 1 minute. Add the clams and broth and cook for about 4 minutes. Add the shrimp and sprinkle with salt and black pepper before cooking for about 2 minutes.
2. Stir in the lime juice and zucchini and cook for 2 to 3 minutes. Garnish with the parsley and serve.

Zucchini with Scallops

In this dish spiralized zucchini is prepared with sweet scallops, and finished with the tangy hit of fresh lemon zest and scallion. This is a perfect family meal!

MAKES: 4 servings
PREPARATION TIME: 15 minutes
COOKING TIME: 10 minutes

2 tablespoons Extra Virgin Olive Oil

2 Garlic Cloves, minced

4 large Zucchinis, spiralized

Sea Salt, to taste

Freshly Ground Black Pepper, to taste

1 pound Bay Scallops, cleaned and rinsed

½ tablespoon Fresh Lemon juice

½ cup Scallions, chopped

1 teaspoon Lemon Zest, freshly grated

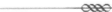

Directions

1. In a large skillet heat 1 tablespoon of the oil on a medium heat. Sauté the garlic for about 1 minute.

Stir in the zucchini, black pepper and salt and cook for 4 to 5 minutes.

2. In another skillet, heat the remaining oil on a medium-high heat. Add the scallops and cook for about 4 minutes, turning once after 2 minutes. Transfer the scallops and the lemon juice into the other skillet with the zucchini and toss to coat well. Garnish with the scallions and lemon zest before serving hot.

Mussels Pasta Deluxe

This is a spiralized zucchini recipe with the great tastes of mussels and cherry tomatoes. This delicious dish is also extremely healthy.

MAKES: 4 servings
PREPARATION TIME: 15 minutes
COOKING TIME: 17 minutes

3 tablespoons Extra Virgin Olive Oil

1 medium White Onion, chopped

2 Celery Stalks, chopped

2 Garlic Cloves, minced

¼ teaspoon Red Pepper Flakes, crushed

2 cups Cherry Tomatoes, halved

2 tablespoons Fresh Thyme, chopped

Sea Salt, to taste

Freshly Ground Black Pepper, to taste

24 Mussels, scrubbed and debearded

4 medium Zucchinis, spiralized

Directions

1. In a large skillet, heat 2 tablespoons of the oil on a medium heat. Add the onion and celery and sauté for 3 to 4 minutes. Add the garlic and red pepper flakes and sauté for about 1 minute before increasing the heat to medium-high. Add the tomatoes, thyme, salt and black pepper. Cover and cook for about 5 minutes before reducing the heat to medium-low and stirring in the mussels. Cover and cook for a further 2 minutes.

2. In another skillet, heat the remaining oil on a medium-high heat. Stir in the zucchini, salt and black pepper, and cook for 4 to 5 minutes. Transfer the zucchini onto a serving plate, top with the mussel mixture and serve.

Zucchini Lobster Bay

*This is a festive dish which is perfect for summertime celebrations.
Enjoy this delicious dish with family and friends.*

MAKES: 2 servings
PREPARATION TIME: 15 minutes
COOKING TIME: 37 minutes

1½ tablespoons Extra Virgin Olive Oil

2 (4-ounce) Lobster Tails, shelled and cut into bite size pieces

1 tablespoon Onion, minced

2 Garlic Cloves, minced

¼ teaspoon Red Pepper Flakes, crushed

2 cups Fresh Tomatoes, finely chopped

1 cup Homemade Vegetable Broth

Sea Salt, to taste

Freshly Ground Black Pepper, to taste

2 medium Zucchinis, spiralized

2 tablespoons minced Cilantro Leaves

Directions

1. In a large skillet, heat 1 tablespoon of the oil on a medium heat. Add the lobster and cook for 5 to 7 minutes. Transfer the lobster into a bowl. In the same skillet, heat the remaining oil on a medium heat. Sauté the onion for 2 minutes before adding the garlic and red pepper flakes and sautéing for an additional minute. Add the tomatoes to the skillet and cook, stirring, for a further 2 minutes.

2. Add the broth, salt and black pepper and bring to a boil before reducing the heat and simmering for 15 to 20 minutes. Stir in the zucchini and lobster and cook for 5 minutes on a medium-low heat. Garnish with the cilantro and serve hot.

8

SAUCE RECIPES

Zucchini Salad with Vegetable Sauce

This is an amazing salad recipe for the whole family. This dish will get any fussy kid to eat fresh vegetables in a delicious meal.

MAKES: 2 servings
PREPARATION TIME: 15 minutes

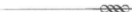

1 cup Plum Tomatoes, chopped

2 small Red Bell Peppers, seeded and chopped

¼ cup Basil Leaves, freshly chopped

1 tablespoon Extra Virgin Olive Oil

2 teaspoons Fresh Lemon juice

½ teaspoon Raw Honey

⅛ teaspoon Dried Thyme, crushed

Sea Salt, to taste

Freshly Ground Black Pepper, to taste

1 large Zucchini, spiralized

Directions

1. Apart for the zucchini, add all of the ingredients into a blender and pulse until smooth.
2. Place the zucchini in a large serving bowl. Add the sauce and mix well before serving immediately.

Zucchini Salad with Mango Sauce

This is a great and delicious salad, ideal for gatherings of family or friends. The mango with almond butter gives a delicious sweetness to the zucchini.

MAKES: 4 servings
PREPARATION TIME: 10 minutes

1 cup Fresh Mango, peeled, pitted and cubed

½ cup Almond Butter

1 teaspoon Raw Honey

2 teaspoons Fresh Lemon juice

2 large Zucchinis, spiralized

¼ cup Almonds, chopped

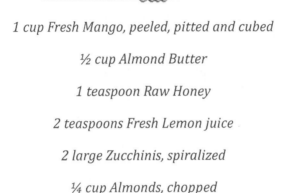

Directions

1. In a blender, add the mango, butter, honey and lemon juice, and pulse until smooth.
2. Place the zucchini in a large serving bowl. Add the sauce and mix well. Top with almonds and serve immediately.

Zucchini Salad with Butter Sauce

This recipe makes a light yet flavorful salad for lunchtime. The wonderfully delicious and creamy sauce with this salad dresses up the zucchini and squash nicely.

MAKES: 2 servings
PREPARATION TIME: 15 minutes

1 medium Zucchini, spiralized

1 medium Yellow Squash, spiralized

1 small Red Bell Pepper, seeded and thinly sliced

1 Garlic Clove, minced

½ teaspoon Fresh Ginger, minced

2 tablespoons Almond Butter

½ tablespoon Coconut Aminos

1 tablespoon Fresh Lime juice

½ tablespoon Filtered Water

¼ teaspoon Red Chili Powder

Sea Salt, to taste

Freshly Ground Black Pepper, to taste

1 tablespoon Black toasted Sesame Seeds

Directions

1. In a large serving bowl, mix together the bell pepper, yellow squash and zucchini.
2. In another small bowl, beat together the remaining ingredients, except for the sesame seeds. Mix together the sauce and the vegetables. Top with the sesame seeds and serve immediately.

Sweet & Sour Creamy Zucchini Salad

This is a simple yet colorful springtime salad. The sweet and sour sauce in this recipe adds subtle flavors to this fresh vegetable salad.

MAKES: 2 servings
PREPARATION TIME: 20 minutes

For Salad:

1 small Zucchini, spiralized

¼ cup Carrot, peeled and spiralized

¼ cup Cucumber, spiralized

¼ cup Orange Bell Pepper, seeded and thinly sliced

For Sauce:

¼ cup Almond Butter

3 teaspoons Raw Honey

1 small Garlic Clove, minced

½ teaspoon Fresh Thyme, minced

½ teaspoon Fresh Oregano, minced

½ teaspoon Fresh Basil, minced

1 teaspoon Extra Virgin Olive Oil

3 teaspoons Fresh Lemon juice

Pinch of Sea Salt

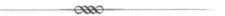

Directions

1. Mix together all of the salad ingredients in a large serving bowl.
2. In another large serving bowl, beat together all of the sauce ingredients. Mix the sauce with the vegetable salad before serving immediately.

Creamy Steamed Zucchini

This delicious salad is filling, healthy and light. This dish is ideal for a lunchtime table.

MAKES: 2 servings
PREPARATION TIME: 15 minutes
COOKING TIME: 8 minutes

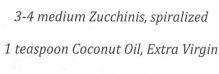

3-4 medium Zucchinis, spiralized

1 teaspoon Coconut Oil, Extra Virgin

1 cup White Onion

2 Garlic Cloves, minced

⅓ cup Unsweetened Coconut Milk

Pinch of Red Pepper Flakes, crushed

Sea Salt, to taste

Freshly Ground Black Pepper, to taste

1 Scallion, chopped

Directions

1. Arrange a steamer basket over a pan of boiling water. Place the zucchini in the steamer basket,

cover and steam for about 2 minutes. Drain well and transfer the zucchini into a serving bowl.

2. In a skillet, heat the oil on a medium heat. Sauté the onion for 4 to 5 minutes before adding the garlic and sautéing for 1 minute. Remove the skillet from the heat and let the mixture cool slightly. In a blender, add the onion mixture, coconut milk and seasoning, and pulse until smooth. Pour the sauce over the steamed zucchini and gently toss to coat well. Garnish with the scallions before serving immediately.

Sautéed Zucchini in Avocado Sauce

This is a super quick, easy and healthy sautéed zucchini meal with a delicious creamy sauce. This recipe prepares a perfect vegetarian dish ideal for the summer months.

MAKES: 2 servings
PREPARATION TIME: 15 minutes
COOKING TIME: 6 minutes

2 tablespoons Extra Virgin Olive Oil

2 Garlic Clove, minced and divided in half

1 large Zucchini, spiralized

2 Avocados, peeled and pitted

½ tablespoon Fresh Lemon Juice

Sea Salt, to taste

Freshly Ground Black Pepper, to taste

Directions

1. In a large skillet, heat 1 tablespoon of the oil on a medium-high heat. Sauté half of the garlic clove for 1 minute. Add the zucchini and sauté for 4 to 5

minutes. Transfer the mixture into a large serving bowl.

2. In another bowl, add the remaining oil, garlic, avocados, lemon juice and seasoning and mash until creamy. Place the avocado sauce over the zucchini mixture and serve.

Spicy Zucchini Fix

This is a tasty zucchini dish with a mild spicy tomato sauce. The combination of the spicy sauce and zucchini work wonderfully well together in this dish.

MAKES: 2 servings
PREPARATION TIME: 15 minutes
COOKING TIME: 27 minutes

---

1 tablespoon Extra Virgin Olive Oil

½ cup White Onion, chopped

1 tablespoon Garlic, minced

1½ cups Fresh Tomatoes, finely chopped

1 cup Filtered Water

¼ teaspoon Ground Cumin

⅛ teaspoon Cayenne Pepper

Sea Salt, to taste

Freshly Ground Black Pepper, to taste

2 tablespoons Fresh Thyme, chopped

3 medium Zucchinis, spiralized

Directions

1. In a large skillet, heat the oil on a medium-high heat. Sauté the onion for 4 to 5 minutes before adding the garlic and sautéing for a further minute. Add the chopped tomatoes and cook, stirring, for 3 to 4 minutes. Add the water and spices and bring to a boil. Reduce the heat and, whilst stirring occasionally, simmer for 10 to 15 minutes, or until cooked to your satisfaction.
2. Stir in the thyme and zucchini and cook for a further 2-3 minutes before serving hot.

9

HOLIDAY RECIPES

Zucchini & Cranberry Salad

This is a wonderfully fresh salad that has a fruity and nutty flavor. The combination of crunchy walnuts, sticky sweet cranberries and the mild tangy dressing gives the zucchini a superb flavor.

MAKES: 2 servings
PREPARATION TIME: 15 minutes

For Salad:

2 medium Zucchinis, spiralized

4 cups Romaine Lettuce, torn

½ cup Fresh Cranberries

1 tablespoon Mint Leaves, freshly chopped

¼ cup *Walnuts, toasted and chopped*

For Dressing:

1 tablespoon *Extra Virgin Olive Oil*

1 tablespoon *Fresh Lime juice*

½ tablespoon *Raw Honey*

Sea Salt, to taste

Freshly Ground Black Pepper, to taste

Directions

1. In a large serving bowl, mix together all of the salad ingredients, except for the walnuts. In another bowl, mix together all of the dressing ingredients before pouring the dressing over the salad and gently tossing to mix well.
2. Garnish with the walnuts and serve immediately.

Rainbow Zucchini Salad

This is a bright and beautifully colorful salad that is full of vegetables, fruit and fresh herbs. The use of avocado gives a refreshing creaminess to this salad.

MAKES: 4 servings
PREPARATION TIME: 20 minutes

---

1 medium Zucchini, spiralized

1 medium Carrot, peeled and spiralized

1 small Apple, cored and chopped

1 small Pear, cored and chopped

½ small Yellow Bell Pepper, seeded and sliced thinly

½ Orange Bell Pepper, seeded and sliced thinly

1 small Red Onion, chopped

1 small Avocado, peeled, pitted and cubed

2 tablespoons minced Cilantro Leaves

2 tablespoons Mint Leaves, freshly chopped

Sea Salt, to taste

Freshly Ground Black Pepper, to taste

2 tablespoons Fresh Lemon juice

Directions

1. In a large serving bowl, mix together all of the salad ingredients and toss to coat well.
2. Serve immediately.

Spiced Zucchini Tomato Soup

This is one simple yet richly flavorful soup. You will love this soup until the last spoon from the soup bowl.

MAKES: 4 servings
PREPARATION TIME: 10 minutes
COOKING TIME: 25 minutes

1 tablespoon Extra Virgin Coconut Oil

1 large Yellow Onion, chopped

1 teaspoon Dried Basil, crushed

½ teaspoon Ground Cumin

⅛ teaspoon Turmeric Powder

½ teaspoon Red Pepper Flakes, crushed

3 cups Fresh Tomatoes, chopped

2 cups Homemade Vegetable Broth

1½ cups Unsweetened Coconut Milk

Sea Salt, to taste

Freshly Ground Black Pepper, to taste

2 tablespoon Fresh Lime juice

3 medium Zucchinis, spiralized

1 teaspoon Lime Zest, freshly grated

Directions

1. In a large soup pan, heat the oil on a medium heat. Sauté the onion for 3 to 4 minutes. Add the basil and spices and sauté for 1 minute. Add the tomatoes and cook for 1 to 2 minutes whilst crushing with the back of the spoon. Add the broth and bring to a boil on high heat. Reduce the heat and simmer, covered, for about 10 minutes. Stir in the coconut milk and simmer for a further 5 minutes. Remove the pan from the heat and cool slightly. In a blender, add the soup and pulse in batches until smooth.

2. Return the soup to the pan. Cook for 2 to 3 minutes, or until heated through. Stir in the salt, black pepper and lime juice and remove from the heat. Place the spiralized zucchini in serving bowls and pour over the hot soup. Garnish with lime zest and serve immediately.

Zucchini & Chicken Soup

This is a purely comforting, filing and delicious soup. This dish will help you fight against the cold winter nights.

MAKES: 4 servings
PREPARATION TIME: 15 minutes
COOKING TIME: 6 hours

---

3 tablespoons Extra Virgin Olive Oil

1 cup White Onion, chopped

3 Celery Stalks, chopped

2 small Carrots, peeled and chopped

2 Garlic Cloves minced

1 teaspoon Dried Thyme, minced

½ teaspoon Red Pepper Flakes, crushed

½ teaspoon Ground Cumin

¼ teaspoon Ground Cilantro

Sea Salt, to taste

Freshly Ground Black Pepper, to taste

4 Grass-Fed boneless Chicken Thighs

4 cups Homemade Chicken Broth

3 medium Zucchinis

½ cup freshly chopped Parsley Leaves

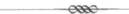

Directions

1. In a large skillet, heat the oil on a medium heat. Sauté the onion, celery and carrots for about 4 minutes. Add the garlic, thyme and spices and sauté for 1 minute. Transfer the mixture into a slow cooker. Dice the chicken thighs and add to the slow cooker with the broth. Set the cooker on low, cover and cook for about 5½ hours.
2. Uncover and stir in the zucchini. Cover and cook for a further 30 minutes. Garnish with the parsley and serve hot.

Zucchini & Sweet Potato Patties

This is a healthy and clever way to get your kids to eat vegetables without any hesitation. These patties are a great hit for weekend meals.

MAKES: 4 servings
PREPARATION TIME: 20 minutes
COOKING TIME: 40 minutes

1 large Organic Egg

¼ teaspoon Ground Cumin

½ teaspoon Red Pepper Flakes, crushed

Sea Salt, to taste

Freshly Ground Black Pepper, to taste

¼ cup Almond Butter, melted

2 tablespoons Almond Flour

1 large Zucchini, spiralized and chopped

1 large Sweet Potato, spiralized and chopped

2 tablespoons minced Cilantro Leaves

Directions

1. Preheat the oven to 375 degrees F and line 2 baking sheets with greased parchment paper.
2. In a large bowl, beat together the egg and spices. Add the butter and flour and mix until combined. Mix in the remaining ingredients. Take ½ cup of the mixture and place into the prepared baking sheet, shaping it like a patty. Repeat with the remaining mixture and arrange on both baking sheets in a single row.
3. Bake for about 10 minutes before reducing the temperature of the oven to 350 degrees F. Bake for a further 15 minutes. Carefully turn the patties and bake for 15 minutes more.

Zucchini with Roasted Tomatoes

The roasted cherry tomatoes in this dish are vibrant, juicy and full of tart flavors. They make a delicious combination with the sautéed zucchini, an ideal combination for a delicious lunch dish.

MAKES: 2 servings
PREPARATION TIME: 20 minutes
COOKING TIME: 20 minutes

2 cups Cherry Tomatoes

3 tablespoons Extra Virgin Olive Oil

2 tablespoons Fresh Lemon Juice

Sea Salt, to taste

Freshly Ground Black Pepper, to taste

2 Garlic Cloves, minced

1 Jalapeño Pepper, seeded and chopped

2 large Zucchinis, spiralized

2 tablespoons Basil, freshly chopped

Directions

1. Preheat the oven to 400 degrees F and grease a roasting pan. In a large bowl, mix together the

tomatoes, 1 tablespoon of the oil, lemon juice, salt and black pepper. Transfer the tomato mixture into the roasting pan and roast for about 20 minutes.

2. Meanwhile, in a large skillet, heat the remaining oil on a medium heat. Sauté the garlic and jalapeño pepper for 1 minute. Add the zucchini, salt and black pepper and cook for 3 to 4 minutes. Transfer the zucchini mixture onto a serving plate. Top with the roasted tomatoes, garnish with the basil and serve hot.

Zucchini with Prawns

This is a super quick zucchini recipe which is really delightful, flavorful and healthy. A perfect combination with prawns!

MAKES: 2 servings
PREPARATION TIME: 20 minutes (plus time to marinate)
COOKING TIME: 8 minutes

---

3 Garlic Cloves, minced

¼ teaspoon Fresh Ginger, minced

1 teaspoon Coconut Aminos

1 teaspoon Raw Honey

½ teaspoon Red Pepper Flakes, crushed

12 Fresh King Prawns, peeled and deveined

3 tablespoons Coconut Oil, Extra Virgin

2 large Zucchinis, spiralized

Sea Salt, to taste

Freshly Ground Black Pepper, to taste

1 tablespoon Fresh Lemon juice

2 tablespoons Parsley, freshly chopped

Directions

1. In a large bowl, mix together 2 minced garlic cloves, ginger, coconut aminos, honey and ¼ teaspoon of red pepper flakes. Add the prawns and generously coat with the marinade before covering refrigerating for at least 2 to 3 hours. In a large skillet, heat 2 tablespoons of oil on a medium heat and add the prawns and marinade. Stir fry for 2 to 4 minutes before removing from the heat and keeping warm.

2. In another large skillet, heat the remaining oil on a medium heat. Add the remaining garlic and sauté for 1 minute. Add the zucchini, remaining red pepper flakes, salt and black pepper and cook for 2 to 3 minutes. Stir in the lemon juice and remove from the heat.

3. Transfer the zucchini mixture onto a serving plate. Top with the prawns, garnish with the parsley and serve hot.

Zucchini with Sardines

Grilled sardines and sautéed zucchini makes a perfect combination for a special dinner party. This is also a fantastic recipe to be enjoyed by the whole family for a special occasion.

MAKES: 4 servings
PREPARATION TIME: 20 minutes
COOKING TIME: 10 minutes

For Sardines:

8 medium Whole Fresh Sardines, gutted, rinsed and dried

1½ tablespoons Extra Virgin Olive Oil

2 tablespoons Fresh Lemon juice

Sea Salt, to taste

Freshly Ground Black Pepper, to taste

For Zucchini:

1 tablespoon Extra Virgin Olive Oil

1 Garlic Clove, minced

1 Jalapeño Pepper, seeded and chopped

3 large Zucchinis, spiralized

Sea Salt, to taste

Freshly Ground Black Pepper, to taste

1 tablespoon Fresh Lemon juice

1 teaspoon Lemon Zest, freshly grated

Directions

1. Preheat the grill to a medium-high heat and grease the grill grate. Place the sardines in a large baking dish. Drizzle with the oil and lemon juice and sprinkle with the salt and black pepper. Grill for about 5 minutes, turning once after 2½ minutes. Transfer the sardines into a large dish and cover with foil to keep them warm.
2. For the zucchini, in a large skillet heat the oil on a medium heat. Sauté the garlic and jalapeño pepper for 1 minute. Add the zucchini, salt and black pepper and cook for 3 to 4 minutes. Stir in the lemon juice and remove from the heat.
3. Transfer the zucchini mixture onto serving plates. Place the sardines alongside the zucchini, garnish with the lemon zest and serve.

Creamy Zucchini Casserole

This recipe is an easy way to prepare a tasty and healthy casserole. This dish tastes so good, even those who do not like the taste of zucchini may love to enjoy this tasty meal.

MAKES: 4 servings
PREPARATION TIME: 20 minutes
COOKING TIME: 50 minutes

4 large Organic Eggs

2 tablespoons Coconut Cream

1 tablespoon Extra Virgin Coconut Oil

¼ cup Almond Meal

Sea Salt, to taste

Freshly Ground Black Pepper, to taste

4 cups Zucchini, spiralized

1 scallion, sliced thinly

Directions

1. Preheat the oven to 300 degrees F and grease an 8x8-inch baking dish.
2. In a large bowl, beat together the eggs, cream, oil, 3

tablespoons of almond meal, salt and black pepper. Stir in the zucchini. Place ⅓ of the zucchini noodles into the prepared baking dish. Place ⅓ of the scallions over the noodles. Repeat the layers twice more. Pour any remaining egg mixture from the bowl over the layers and evenly sprinkle with the almond meal.

3. Bake for about 50 minutes, or until cooked.

Baked Zucchini & Meatballs

The zucchini and meatballs recipe make a wonderful combination in this baked dish. This recipe offers a delicious and flavorful dinner for family and friends.

MAKES: 4 servings
PREPARATION TIME: 20 minutes
COOKING TIME: 40 minutes

For Meatballs:

1 pound Grass-Fed Lean Ground Beef

1 Garlic Clove, minced

2 tablespoons minced Cilantro Leaves

½ teaspoon Ground Cilantro

1 teaspoon Ground Cumin

1 teaspoon Cayenne Pepper

Sea Salt, to taste

Freshly Ground Black Pepper, to taste

For Zucchini:

2 tablespoons Extra Virgin Olive Oil

1 White Onion, chopped

2 Garlic Cloves, minced

½ teaspoon Ground Cilantro

½ teaspoon Ground Cumin

1 teaspoon Cayenne Pepper

Sea Salt, to taste

Freshly Ground Black Pepper, to taste

2 cups Tomatoes, chopped finely

4 small Zucchinis, spiralized

Directions

1. Preheat the oven to 350 degrees F.
2. In a large bowl, mix together all of the meatball ingredients. Make your desired sized balls from the mixture before setting aside. In a large oven proof skillet, heat the oil on medium heat. Sauté the onion for 4 to 5 minutes. Add the garlic and spices and sauté for 1 minute. Add the tomatoes and zucchini and cook for 3 to 4 minutes more.
3. Remove from the heat, add the meatballs and gently press into the zucchini mixture. Transfer the skillet into the oven and bake for 25 to 30 minutes.

10

VARIETY DISHES

Nutty Zucchini & Mixed Berry Salad

This is a filling, refreshing and delicious salad with a crunchy and nutty texture. This salad will be a great hit for lunch or for a light dinner.

MAKES: 4 servings
PREPARATION TIME: 10 minutes

1 large Zucchini, spiralized

1 large Carrot, peeled and spiralized

½ cup Fresh Strawberries, hulled and sliced

¼ cup Fresh Raspberries

¼ cup Fresh Blueberries

¼ cup Fresh Blackberries

2 cups Fresh Baby Spinach

½ cup Golden Raisins

½ cup Almonds, toasted and chopped

1 tablespoon Extra Virgin Olive Oil

2 tablespoons Fresh Lime juice

Sea Salt, to taste

Freshly Ground Black Pepper, to taste

¼ cup Mint Leaves, freshly chopped

Directions

1. In a large serving bowl, except for the mint, mix together all of the ingredients.
2. Garnish with the mint and serve immediately.

Zucchini, Apple & Pomegranate Mi

This is a tempting salad which is easy to throw together. This delicious and healthy salad is good for the whole family.

MAKES: 2 servings
PREPARATION TIME: 15 minutes

For Salad:

2 medium Zucchinis, spiralized

1 large Apple, cored and chopped

3 tablespoons Fresh Pomegranate Seeds

2 tablespoons Fresh Mint Leaves, chopped

2 tablespoons Walnuts, chopped

For Dressing:
¼ cup Fresh Pomegranate juice

1 teaspoon Organic Honey

2 tablespoons Fresh Lemon juice

1 tablespoon Extra Virgin Olive Oil

Sea Salt, to taste

Freshly Ground Black Pepper, to taste

Directions

1. In a large serving bowl, mix together the zucchini, apple and pomegranate seeds. In another bowl, mix together all of the dressing ingredients before pouring the dressing over the salad. Ensure it is mixed well with the dressing.
2. Garnish with the mint and walnuts, and serve immediately.

Chilled Zucchini Soup

This recipe makes a delicious vegetable soup with a creamy and silky texture without using any dairy products. This dish is great for a summer lunch or a light supper.

MAKES: 4 servings
PREPARATION TIME: 15 minutes (plus time to chill)
COOKING TIME: 30 minutes

---

2 tablespoons Coconut Oil, Extra Virgin

1 small White Onion, chopped

2 small Garlic Cloves, minced

1 teaspoon Dried Thyme, crushed

¼ teaspoon Red Pepper Flakes, crushed

2 large Zucchinis, chopped

Sea Salt, to taste

Freshly Ground Black Pepper, to taste

⅔ cup Homemade Vegetable Broth

1½ cups Filtered Water

1 small Zucchini, spiralized

Directions

1. In a large soup pan, heat the oil on a medium heat. Sauté the onion for 8 to 9 minutes before adding the garlic, thyme and red pepper flakes and sautéing for 1 minute more. Add the chopped large zucchinis, salt and black pepper and cook, stirring occasionally, for 8 to 10 minutes. Add the broth and water and bring to a boil on a high heat. Reduce the heat and simmer for about 10 minutes. Remove the soup pan from the heat and let the liquid cool slightly.
2. In a blender, add the soup and pulse in batches until smooth. Transfer the soup into a large bowl and season with salt and black pepper. Cover and refrigerate to chill before topping with the small spiralized zucchini and serving.

Zucchini & Shrimp Soup

This is one of the quickest and easiest soups. The combination of shrimp and zucchini works well for this hearty soup.

MAKES: 4 servings
PREPARATION TIME: 15 minutes
COOKING TIME: 5 minutes

2 cups Homemade Chicken Broth

1¾ cups Unsweetened Coconut Milk

½ teaspoon Fresh Ginger, grated

1 pound Shrimp, peeled and deveined

1 large Zucchini, spiralized

2 tablespoons Fresh Lime juice

Sea Salt, to taste

Freshly Ground Black Pepper, to taste

3 tablespoons minced Cilantro Leaves

Directions

1. In a large soup pan, add the broth and coconut milk and bring to a boil on medium-high heat. Reduce

the heat and add the ginger, shrimp and zucchini and simmer for 4 to 5 minutes.

2. Stir in lime juice, salt and black pepper and remove from the heat. Garnish with the cilantro and serve hot.

Zucchini & Bell Pepper Wraps

This fresh vegetable wrap is perfect for lunchboxes, picnics or as a light meal. The use of the refreshing and cooling basil pesto adds a delicious touch to these wraps.

MAKES: 4 servings
PREPARATION TIME: 20 minutes

For Pesto:

2 cups Fresh Basil Leaves

2 large Garlic Cloves, chopped

⅓ cup Cashew nuts

½ cup Extra Virgin Olive Oil

Sea Salt, to taste

Freshly Ground Black Pepper, to taste

For Wraps:

1 medium Zucchini, spiralized and chopped

1 small Carrot, peeled, spiralized and chopped

1 Orange Bell Pepper, seeded and thinly sliced

1 Red Bell Pepper, seeded and thinly sliced

½ medium Avocado, peeled, pitted and thinly sliced

4 large Kale Leaves, trimmed

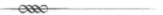

Directions

1. For the pesto, add all of the pesto ingredients into a blender and pulse until smooth. Transfer the pesto into a bowl and refrigerate before serving.
2. In a bowl, mix together the zucchini, carrot, bell peppers and avocado. Place a kale leaf on a large plate and arrange ¼ of the zucchini mixture over the leaf. Top with ¼ of the pesto. Roll the leaves around the zucchini mixture before repeating with the remaining leaves, zucchini mixture and pesto.

Zucchini Buns & Chicken Sandwich

This recipe is a fun way to make a creative dish for a light lunch or a snack. These sandwiches are so delicious that your kids will ask for more!

MAKES: 2 servings
PREPARATION TIME: 15 minutes (plus time to refrigerate)
COOKING TIME: 10 minutes

For Buns:

2 tablespoons Extra Virgin Olive Oil

2 Garlic Cloves, minced

3 large Zucchinis, spiralized

Sea Salt, to taste

Freshly Ground Black Pepper, to taste

2 large Organic Eggs, beaten

2 Organic Egg Whites, beaten

For Avocado Mash:

1 Avocado, peeled, pitted and chopped

1½ tablespoons freshly minced Parsley Leaves

Pinch of Sea Salt

Pinch of Red Pepper Flakes, crushed

For Sandwiches:
2 Red Onion Slices

2 large Tomato Slices

4-ounce Grass-Fed cooked, chopped Chicken Breast

2 Romaine Lettuce Leaves, torn

Directions

1. In a large skillet, heat 1 tablespoon of the oil on a medium heat. Sauté the garlic for 1 minute. Add the zucchini and sprinkle with salt and black pepper, and cook for 3 to 4 minutes. Transfer the zucchini mixture into a bowl. Immediately mix in the beaten eggs and the egg whites. Transfer the mixture into 4 large ramekins, filling half full. Cover the ramekins with wax paper and place a weight over the wax paper to press down firmly. Refrigerate for at least 20 minutes. In a large skillet, heat the remaining oil on a medium-low heat. Carefully transfer the zucchini buns into the skillet and cook for 2 to 3 minutes. Change the side and cook for 2 to 3 minutes more. Transfer the buns onto a plate.
2. Meanwhile, add all of the avocado mash ingredients into a bowl. With a fork, mash till smooth and creamy, and then set aside. Preheat the grill to a medium heat and grease the grill grate. Grill the onion slices for 2 minutes, turning after 1 minute.

Grill the tomato slices for 30 seconds each side.

3. Place one bun onto a serving plate and spread the avocado mash over the bun. Place 1 onion slice over the avocado mash and place half of the chicken over the onion. Top with the tomato slice and half of the torn lettuce. Cover with other the bun. Repeat with the remaining buns.

Zucchini & Sweet Potato Waffles

This is a flavorful breakfast recipe. The zucchini and sweet potato makes a wonderful combination with the other ingredients used for this dish.

MAKES: 2 servings
PREPARATION TIME: 15 minutes
COOKING TIME: 10 minutes

2 small Zucchinis, spiralized, chopped and squeezed

½ pound Sweet Potato, peeled, spiralized, chopped and squeezed

½ small Red Onion, finely chopped

2 Garlic Cloves, minced

1 tablespoon Fresh Parsley, minced

¼ teaspoon Cayenne Pepper

Sea Salt, to taste

Freshly Ground Black Pepper, to taste

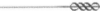

Directions

1. Grease a preheated waffle iron before cooking.
2. In a large bowl, mix together all of the ingredients. Place the zucchini mixture into the preheated waffle iron. Cook for 8 to 10 minutes, or until golden brown and crispy.

Spicy Zucchini & Carrot Loaf Cake

This savory vegetable loaf cake is packed with zucchini and carrots. This cake is great for breakfast or as a snack.

MAKES: 4 servings
PREPARATION TIME: 15 minutes
COOKING TIME: 55 minutes

2 tablespoons Coconut Oil, Extra Virgin

2 Garlic Cloves, minced

1 Jalapeño Pepper, chopped

4 medium Zucchinis, spiralized and chopped

4 medium Carrots, peeled, spiralized and chopped

¼ teaspoon Red Pepper Flakes, crushed

Sea Salt, to taste

Freshly Ground Black Pepper, to taste

¼ cup Coconut Flour

½ teaspoon Baking Powder

6 large Organic Eggs

¼ cup Unsweetened Coconut Milk

2 tablespoons minced Cilantro Leaves

Directions

1. Preheat the oven to 350 degrees F and line a loaf pan with parchment paper.
2. In a skillet, heat the oil on a medium heat. Sauté the garlic and jalapeño pepper for about 1 minute. Add the zucchini, carrot, red pepper flakes, salt and black pepper and cook for 8 to 9 minutes. Remove the pan from the heat and let it cool.
3. In a bowl, mix together the flour, baking powder and a pinch of salt. In another bowl, beat together the eggs and coconut milk. Fold the egg mixture into the flour mixture. Fold in the zucchini mixture and cilantro. Transfer the mixture into the prepared loaf pan. Bake for about 40 to 45 minutes. The cake is ready when a toothpick inserted into the center comes out clean.

Zucchini Pancakes

This is an awesome recipe for pancakes! The zucchini marries nicely with the flour, eggs and honey for mild, sweet and delicious pancakes.

MAKES: 4 servings
PREPARATION TIME: 15 minutes
COOKING TIME: 4 minutes

½ cup Almond Flour

1 tablespoon Flax Meal

⅓ teaspoon Baking Soda

Pinch of Sea Salt

1 Organic Egg, separated

½ tablespoon Organic Honey

1 tablespoon Coconut Oil, Extra Virgin

½ cup Unsweetened Almond Milk

½ cup Zucchini, spiralized and chopped

Directions

1. Grease a preheated griddle before cooking.
2. In a large bowl, mix together the flour, flax meal,

baking soda and salt. In another bowl, beat together the egg yolk, honey, oil and milk. Mix the honey mixture into the flour mixture. In a small bowl, add the egg white and beat until soft peaks form. Fold the beaten egg white into the flour mixture before folding in the zucchini.

3. Place ¼ cup of the mixture in the griddle and cook for 1 to 2 minutes each side. Make more pancakes by repeating with the remaining mixture.

Zucchini, Chicken & Olive Pizza

This is an easy, delicious and healthy homemade pizza recipe. This pizza may quickly become a firm favorite for everyone in the family, including any fussy eaters.

MAKES: 4 servings
PREPARATION TIME: 20 minutes
COOKING TIME: 27 minutes

For Crust:

1½ cups Almond Meal

1 cup Coconut Flour

1 cup Tapioca Flour

1½ teaspoons Baking Powder

Pinch of Sea Salt

5 Organic Eggs

5 tablespoons Extra Virgin Olive Oil

1 cup Filtered Water

2 Garlic Cloves, minced

1 tablespoon Fresh Rosemary, minced

For Tomato Sauce:

2 cups Fresh Tomatoes, chopped

1 tablespoon Basil Leaves, freshly chopped

1 tablespoon Extra Virgin Olive Oil

1 tablespoon Fresh Lemon juice

Sea Salt, to taste

Freshly Ground Black Pepper, to taste

For Topping:

1 cup Cooked Chicken, cubed

1 medium Zucchini, spiralized and chopped

8-10 Black Olives, pitted and sliced

Pinch of Red Pepper Flakes, crushed

Pinch of Sea Salt

Directions

1. Preheat the oven to 350 degrees F. Grease a pizza pan and line with parchment paper.
2. For the crust, mix together the almond meal, flours, baking powder and salt in a bowl. In a separate bowl, beat together the water, oil and eggs. Mix the egg mixture into the flour mixture. Fold in the garlic and rosemary and mix until a dough forms. Place the dough into the prepared pan and bake for about 15 minutes. Remove from the oven and let it cool slightly. Carefully remove the parchment paper from

underneath the crust.

3. Meanwhile, for the tomato sauce, add all of the sauce ingredients into a blender and pulse until smooth. Spread the tomato sauce evenly over crust. Place the chicken and zucchini over the tomato sauce, and place the olives over the zucchini. Sprinkle with red pepper flakes and salt and bake for 10 to 12 minutes.

11

INGREDIENT SUBSTITIONS

F or some reason or another, you may want to still enjoy these recipes without using gluten-free ingredients. In such cases, here follows some ingredient substitutions that could help you to experience a fulfilled cooking adventure with these recipes. In addition to these suggestions, you may also consider tweaking these recipes with your own list of favorite ingredients wherever possible.

1. **Oil:** You may substitute extra virgin coconut oil or extra virgin olive oil with sunflower oil, corn oil, vegetable oil or your favorite cooking oil.
2. **Butter:** You may substitute nut butters with your favorite butter or margarine.
3. **Protein:** You may substitute free-range, wild or grass-fed proteins with regular food store versions.
4. **Flour:** You may substitute almond flour and other nut flours with all-purpose flour or whole wheat flour
5. **Sweetener:** You may substitute coconut sugar, homemade applesauce, raw honey or organic dates

with brown sugar, white/granulated sugar, regular honey or your favorite sweetener.

6. **Seasonings & Spices:** You may substitute coconut vinegar with white vinegar and coconut aminos with soy sauce. You may also substitute sea salt with regular table salt or whichever salt you prefer.

7. **Beverages:** You may substitute unsweetened almond milk and coconut milk with your favorite dairy or non-dairy milk.

12

ZOODLES FOR NOODLES!

Certainly, many would agree that you haven't started your spiralizing journey until you've started to spiralize zucchinis. The overall health benefits of creating tasty spiralized zucchini dishes are remarkable. Additionally, preparing meals with spiralized zucchinis is a welcome inspiration to many home cooks. With this cookbook, you'll be always prepared to make a variety of sumptuous meals that are prepared using the most loved spiralizable vegetable.

When I first got my spiralizer, I was struggling to come up with healthy gluten-free meal ideas for my zucchinis. But I never gave up there. As time went by, I would experiment with different gluten-free ingredients that would help me to easily avoid heavy carbs and gluten. Excitingly, my interest grew as I continued to create new ways to include spiralized zucchinis in my daily gluten-free lifestyle. In the end, by using spiralized zucchinis with other gluten-free combinations, I have continued to experience remarkable health benefits. Now, as a successful gluten-free convert, I have also become an advocate for spiralized zucchinis. I have found that the rewards of including healthy zucchini pasta meals in a gluten-free diet are incalculable.

Thanks again for choosing my spiralized zucchini cookbook. If you have found it to be worthwhile, I would appreciate if you would let other readers know about it. Please join me on a thrilling journey to better health—let's eat zoodles for noodles!

From my kitchen to yours,
Kari James

13

EASY CONVERSION GUIDE

T his spiralized zucchini cookbook is for everyone! Hence, this measurement conversion guide is included to enhance the overall user experience of this recipe book. Particularly, readers who are living in the UK will find this conversion chart to be quite helpful for easily converting any of these recipes.

FOR LIQUID INGREDIENTS

1 teaspoon (tsp) = 6 milliliters (ml)

1 tablespoon (tbsp) = 15 milliliters (ml)

1/8 cup = 30 milliliters (ml)

¼ cup = 60 milliliters (ml)

½ cup = 120 milliliters (ml)

1 cup = 240 milliliters (ml)

FOR DRY OR SOLID INGREDIENTS

1 teaspoon (tsp) = 5 grams (g)

1 tablespoon (tbsp) = 15 grams (g)

1 ounce (oz) = 28 grams (g)

1 cup nut flour or any other gluten-free flour = 150 grams (g)

1 cup coconut sugar = 175 grams (g)

1 cup spiralized fruit or vegetable = 175 grams (g)

1 small spiralized courgette, fruit or other vegetable = 120 -150 grams (g)

1 medium spiralized courgette, fruit or vegetable = 195 -225 grams (g)

1 large spiralized courgette, fruit or vegetable = 250 -315 grams (g)

1 cup nuts or seeds = 200 grams (g)

1/8 cup nut butter = 30 grams (g)

¼ cup nut butter = 55 grams (g)

1/3 cup nut butter = 75 grams (g)

½ cup nut butter = 115 grams (g)

2/3 cup nut butter = 150 grams (g)

¾ cup nut butter = 170 grams (g)

1 cup nut butter = 225 grams (g)

OVEN TEMPERATURES

275° Fahrenheit (F) = 140° Celsius (C) or Gas Mark 1

300° Fahrenheit (F) = 150° Celsius (C) or Gas Mark 2

325° Fahrenheit (F) = 165° Celsius (C) or Gas Mark 3

350° Fahrenheit (F) = 180° Celsius (C) or Gas Mark 4

375° Fahrenheit (F) = 190° Celsius (C) or Gas Mark 5

400° Fahrenheit (F) = 200° Celsius (C) or Gas Mark 6

425° Fahrenheit (F) = 220° Celsius (C) or Gas Mark 7

450° Fahrenheit (F) = 230° Celsius (C) or Gas Mark 8

45127610R00145

Made in the USA
San Bernardino, CA
04 February 2017